Updated Version

Digital Medical Home

HOW THE TELEMEDICINE REVOLUTION
IGNITED THE CREATION OF
PRECISION HEALTH

Jay H. Sanders, MD, FACP
Michael S. Gorton, MS, JD

WITH CONTRIBUTIONS BY

G. Byron Brooks, EE, MD and Michael Brombach, COO

MVHL

Quantity sales special discounts are available on quantity purchases
by corporations, associations, and others. For details, contact the
publisher at carol@markvictorhansenlibrary.com

Orders by U.S. trade bookstores and wholesalers.
Email: carol@markvictorhansenlibrary.com

Creative Contributor - Alaina Gangestad
Cover Design - Low & Joe Creative, Brea, CA 92821
Book Layout - DBree, StoneBear Design

Manufactured and printed in the United States of America distributed
globally by markvictorhansenlibrary.com

MVHL

New York | Los Angeles | London | Sydney

ISBN: 979-8-88581-083-8 Hardback
ISBN: 979-8-88581-084-5 Paperback
ISBN: 979-8-88581-073-9 eBook
Library of Congress Control Number: 2022923186

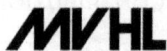

Contents

Dedications-Acknowledgements

by
Michael Gorton, BS MS JD
Recuro - Founder and CEO

When the great Spartan leader, Leonidas, faced an invading army, outnumbered a thousand to one, neither he nor his soldiers fled. Those Spartans lived by a creed whereby they understood the opposite of fear. In the early days of Teladoc, the DEA came into our office with guns and badges. Entrepreneurs must endure many challenges not seen in corporate America, but even the intrepid entrepreneur might cower when faced by circumstances like this. On that day, the 35 (or so) Teladoc employees did not run and hide. Like the Spartans, they knew the opposite of fear is love and passion. You will not run and hide if you believe in love, and are passionate about what is behind you, what you are defending. You stand strong and protect it.

I dedicate this book to those 35 individuals at Teladoc who, in the early years of telemedicine, stood strong, disrupted the system and improved Healthcare. Before Teladoc, a request to see a doctor took days to happen. Now it almost always happens in under ten minutes. The pathway to that outcome was difficult.

For those of you at Recuro, who are working with me on the next journey, the result will be health and longevity.

May We live beyond 600!

Dedications-Acknowledgements

by

Jay H. Sanders, M.D., FACP, FACAAI, FATA

A telecommunication solution introduced in the late 1960s by Dr. Kenneth Bird at the Massachusetts General Hospital initially addressed a traffic problem in Boston. His subsequent realization that this solution had much greater applications in addressing the issues of effective access to healthcare for those who had been disenfranchised from the healthcare delivery system created a revolution in how healthcare could be provided. His idea and commitment, combined with the dramatic advances in telecommunications technology, now affords us the ability to provide healthcare to a person in need anywhere and at any time.

Foreword

by
Bernard A Harris, MD, MBA, FACP
Former NASA Astronaut

I have been involved with Telemedicine in various roles for over 25 years at NASA, Vesalius Ventures and the American Telemedicine Association. I have known these two authors for decades. Jay Sanders and I first met in the 1990s when I was an astronaut, and he was carrying the banner and planting seeds for telemedicine. Michael and I met in the very early days of Teladoc through his co-founder, Byron Brooks and Byron's colleague, Oscar Boultinghouse. In addition, the publisher, Mark Victor Hansen, is a friend who was inducted as a member of the Horatio Alger Association in the same class as me in 2000.

Because of the deep and long-standing connections coupled with my personal knowledge of the industry, I cannot think of two authors better qualified to tell the story of the history of telemedicine. While much of the book tells the sometimes harrowing tales of the development of this industry—the most important part covers *what's next.* These two people have played a pivotal role in telemedicine since its infancy. And each, in their own way, has continued to serve as leaders in the industry today.

I spent my post-astronaut career working with entrepreneurs who were building assets to improve care in this country. I am no stranger to telemedicine. During my Space Shuttle missions, I worked with the Mayo Clinic to conduct the first telemedicine conference from space. And I helped to develop clinical techniques, and inflight diagnostic hardware with the capability to communicate with physicians and researchers on earth. In fact, NASA was one of the early utilizers of telemedicine to monitor crew health in orbit.

Later, I was an advisor and friend to the original founders of Teladoc. I was even in attendance at one of the first Teladoc planning sessions with Gorton, Brooks and Boultinghouse at the Barnes and Noble in Webster, Texas.

Before the Covid pandemic, few people knew the value or nature of telemedicine. Now, most people have used it, and many prefer it over traditional health care delivery. The reasoning is simple. It is convenient, less expensive, and improves patient outcomes.

But few people know that the idea began in the summer of 1967 at Massachusetts General Hospital. This remarkable story will be shared in the following pages of this book. More than forty years have passed between 1967 and Teladoc signing its millionth member in December of 2007. This great new idea in the form of Teladoc was finally recognized by MIT Technology Review in 2015 as one of the "Smartest Companies in the World."

The authors will tell you why it took so long, and when you read the stories, you will wonder how they prevailed. The battle was a tough one, even for entrepreneurs. As an investor, I am fond of asking founders, "What keeps you up at night?" I think I know what kept Michael Gorton up at night. But he and his team prevailed to create one of the best-known telemedicine companies in the world.

The American healthcare system is in need of change, and these two authors will tell you how they did it once, and why they are doing it again.

Digital Medical Home

A couple of years ago, I (Michael Gorton) called John Halsey to get his opinion on an idea that was brewing in my head about how to use what we built at Teladoc to ignite the next generation of care. When it comes to healthcare, John is one of the most knowledgeable people I know. Generally, he does most of the talking, but that time, he listened. At the end, he said something to the effect, "Sounds like a digital medical home." I loved the term, and with that, we began a journey to once again become disrupters in the healthcare space.

The second person I called was Jay H. Sanders, MD. Over the years, Jay and I have become friends alongside our collegial relationship. Someone once said to us that if Jay is the father of telemedicine, then I am his son. "Dad" and I have had a lot of fun with that one. Last summer, we decided to write this book. It is intended to be a re-telling of the history and challenges, sometimes treacherous and foreboding obstacles to what ultimately became a magnificent telemedicine destination that played a significant role in the pandemic. More importantly, Jay and I recognized that telemedicine should become an efficient delivery tool for the next generation of care.

As Dr. Sanders and I were writing the book, we did not have a title. I thought during the process, one would pop out. Every Tuesday evening, for several months, Jay

Sanders, our ghost writer and transcriber—Alaina Gangestad and I jumped on Zoom to tell stories. By the weekend, Alaina would have the chapter transcribed, and I would work to make it flow.

No titles popped out, so we ran a competition at my company, Recuro Health.

We started with Halsey's Digital Medical Home, which was originally trademarked by Recuro (trademark now removed). I couldn't shake it, but the title was not complete. Patty Ward and Jon O'Toole brought the title together by adding the right words for a subtitle.

As you navigate the stories in this book, the title will make sense. The last chapter really pulls it all together and shows how the Digital Medical Home will become a fundamental part of the future of a new kind of preemptive care, designed to catch things before they become dangerous and expensive.

But first, fasten your seatbelt and enjoy the many tales that led to the Telemedicine Revolution . . .

CHAPTER 1

The Traffic in Boston

Everything begins with an idea
— Earl Nightingale

In the Fall of 2002, Nelson woke up, excited about an important and busy day. He was overweight and not terribly healthy, so when he rolled out of bed, and felt something was different, he ignored it. Nelson had become an expert at ignoring health issues. Terry, his wife admonished him and told him to go to the doctor. That was not going to happen. Today's important meeting would change the course of his business, and therefore could not be missed.

During the forty-five-minute drive from home to downtown Dallas, the problem worsened, but only a small amount. He thought it was probably a cold, or something he had eaten the night before. Nelson was always positive, tough, and determined. It was a determination that had painted the pathway of success in his life.

But then things suddenly changed. His vision began to blur, and the situation became catastrophic. Nelson lost control of his pickup truck at 75 miles per hour, and the fatality that occurred next was inevitable.

That scenario is a likely possibility, but it is not what happened on that day. Thirty-seven years earlier, on a hot day in Boston, the butterfly effect, the idea that small things that happened in the past can have non-linear impacts on a complex system, saved Nelson's life.

Here is what really happened.

Nelson woke up, excited about an important and busy day. He was overweight and not terribly healthy, so when he rolled out of bed, and felt something was different, he ignored it. Nelson had become an expert at ignoring health issues. Terry, his wife admonished him and told him to go to the doctor. That was not going to happen. Today's important meeting would change the course of his business, and therefore could not be missed.

As he was pulling out of the driveway that morning, he remembered he was a member of a new healthcare delivery system called Teladoc. He called in the service, and within minutes, Doctor Brooks was on his cell phone asking questions as he drove. As most people often do, Nelson ignored his beloved wife when she suggested he go to the doctor, but he took the advice of Dr. Brooks, who instructed him to drive directly to the ER.

Nelson took Dr. Brooks' advice, and within a few minutes, he was in the local ER. A simple conversation with a physician who could listen, review an electronic medical record, and diagnose, saved Nelson's life.

Dr. Brooks was the co-founder of Teladoc, a company he started because of a seed that pioneer, Jay Sanders, had planted a few years earlier during a speech at the University of Texas Medical Branch in Galveston. This book will tell the sometimes historic, other times startling tales of the road telemedicine took from 1967 Boston to where it is today. Telemedicine has created a new efficiency paradigm in care, and that engine is now on the precipice of an evolution that will revolutionize healthcare into the future. We will tell the complete story in the pages ahead.

First, the butterfly effect from the birth of telemedicine.

The Summer of Love (Jay H. Sanders, M.D.)

The summer of 1967 was explosive: riots, hippies, the Summer of Love, Vietnam, the Beatles, the Stones, and… the birth of telemedicine. Where was I? I was a senior medical resident at Massachusetts General Hospital (MGH) having just returned from two years of studying at the National Institute of Health. In those days, emergency medical specialties didn't exist, and I was running the emergency department (ED). Back then, the senior medical resident and the surgical senior resident would each take two 12-hour shifts running the emergency department. Whoever was on the job, would see each patient that walked through that door and triage them. Every manner of case shows up in the emergency department (ED), so we definitely received intense training.

I remember vividly one particularly hot Boston summer day; I was working my 12-hour shift at the MGH ED, anticipating another traffic injury, chest pain, upper respiratory infection, broken bone, sprain, or abdominal pain. All of these are typical cases in the ED. Instead, the doors burst open and there stood Dr. Kenneth Bird, one of my professors of medicine. Though he was only about five foot seven, he was an imposing effigy. On this day, he was hot, sweaty, red-faced, and clearly upset. I had seen him this way enough times so that no one needed to explain this to me. I knew exactly why he was upset.

You see, the professors of medicine at the Massachusetts General Hospital in those days did not make much of an academic salary—probably no more than $8,000 a year. Many of them were *moonlighting* with their own private practices, and Dr. Bird was one of them. His second job was at Logan Airport where he was the medical director, treating airport employees and sick travelers. Dr. Bird had just come from Logan Airport and anyone who knows Boston knows that Logan Airport and the MGH are not far from each other—3.2 miles to be exact. For clarity, that is just over one mile of tortoise speeds up to and under the Sumner Tunnel, punctuated by over two miles of traffic lights and tourists darting on crowded streets crisscrossed by the historic Freedom Trail. In sum, the drive would burn an hour each way. The round trip was two exhausting hours spent in the car with no cell phone to create value or air conditioner to cool the frustration.

As might be expected, when brilliance is trapped in a place like the Sumner Tunnel with no air conditioning coupled with time management frustration, something great should be conceived. On this day, Dr. Bird burst through the doors of the MGH ED with an idea. We made eye contact, so he charged directly to me with purpose.

"Jay!" He began, grabbing my arm firmly.

I started to say something about how I was sorry he had gotten caught in traffic again, and I know it's so frustrating, the traffic is terrible, yada yada…but he cut me off mid-sentence.

"No, that's not it. I mean, yes, I did get caught in traffic. It is a senseless waste of time, but as I was parked in dead stop traffic under the Sumner and Charles River, I had this idea. What if I purchased two TV cameras and put one here in the ED and one at Logan Airport? I could examine patients over TV and avoid the traffic! What do you think?"

I searched his face for the glimmer of a smile, the whisper of laughter. Was he joking?! He was unsmiling, serious as could be. I thought it was the stupidest idea I had ever heard in my life, but what could I say? I was a resident, and he was my professor.

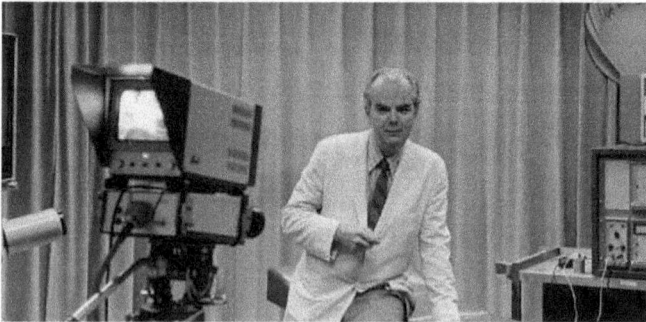

Ken Bird's telemedicine system, circa 1968

I had enough common sense to say simply, "Gee, Dr. Bird! That's a very interesting idea." If necessity is truly the mother of invention, then my professor's necessity was moving with the ferocity of an avalanche.

Being the maverick that he was, Dr. Bird knew another maverick, Dr. John Knowles, who might be able to help him. Dr. Knowles was the general director of MGH. He was, in fact, willing and able to help, and he fed that avalanche by providing Ken with the money to buy those two TV cameras.

In June of 1968, about a year later, I was completing my third year of residency. I took a six-month hematology residency which began in July and was complete by December. Things were progressing with Ken Bird's project and on January 1, 1969, I became the chief medical resident. More importantly, we had a fully functioning telemedicine system operating between the Mass General and Logan Airport Medical Station.

At Logan Airport Medical Station, there was a nurse who would communicate with the various faculty at the Mass General. From the MGH ED, the faculty would assess the patients at Logan Airport and the nurse would treat the patients as needed. What was most remarkable was that, in the late 1960s, most TV cameras were black and white! In addition, the NTSC standard at the time was 240 interlaced scanned lines simulating 480 lines of resolution. Compared with today's TV and monitor resolution, it was TERRIBLE. Even with low resolution and no color, The Chair of Pathology, Dr. Benjamin Castleman and the Chair of Dermatology, Dr. Thomas Fitzpatrick used the system and got so good at interpreting the grayscale that they were basically able to determine the color of a lesion! At this time, my involvement with the telemedicine system was minimal, though I did get to run the first bone marrow sample out to Logan Airport to test if Dr. Castleman could read it from the MGH!

Of course, not everyone was in favor of this new and experimental way of practicing medicine. Dr. Thomas Dwyer, Head of the Department of Psychiatry, was more than skeptical. His words, as I remember them, were, "This system will never work for mental health patients! The special ambiance that exists between the psychiatrist and his or her patients in the room together can never be reproduced by a TV camera!"

Three years later, that same Dr. Dwyer and his faculty wrote a series of articles in the psychiatry literature demonstrating the incredible effectiveness of tele-psychiatry! It turned out that Dr. Dwyer discovered that not only could they reproduce that ambiance, but they could also manipulate it. Just like any movie director would tell you, you can create the emotions of the scene, not only by the dialogue, not only by the facial expressions, but also by how you shoot the scene. When the doctor wanted the patient to see that what they were telling them was important, they would lean in closer to the camera. When the patient didn't seem ready to deal with the emotion of that moment, the doctor would minimize themself by leaning away from the camera. These were things that could not have been done as organically in the office, face-to-face.

The most important thing to note here is that one of telemedicine's biggest naysayers ended up becoming one of its biggest proponents. The stupidest idea I had ever heard in my whole life was gaining traction.

And—spoiler alert—I have been working on that stupid idea ever since!

Who is the Father of Telemedicine?

When I wasn't working at Massachusetts General to complete my residency, I could be found at Regina's Pizzeria, having a coke and some of the best pizza in the world with my friends or wife, talking about many of the crazy and brilliant antics of my professor, Dr. Ken Bird. On a side note, Regina's is so good that I wish I was there eating some of the world's best pizza right now!

Ken, a graduate of Harvard Medical School, specialized in pulmonary diseases. Though he never said it to me directly, I believe he was influenced into this specialty by the fact that in his second year of medical school, he developed tuberculosis and was sent off to Middlesex Sanatorium in Massachusetts, as was the custom in those days. If I remember correctly, he also had a consultative role there after becoming a physician. He may have even been the medical director.

When I was a resident, one of our rotations was to that sanatorium where Ken taught us how to obtain culture specimens from infected patients without the risk of becoming infected. Additionally, he taught us everything else there was to know about tuberculosis. Residents were on-call every other night in those days, so the rotation at the sanatorium was a favorite due to there being few acute situations and, therefore, the ability to get some sleep! I think folks forget that Dr. Bird also researched with a Dr. Harriet Hardy at MIT, and they are both credited with identifying the critical fiber size that causes asbestosis, a chronic lung disease caused by inhaling asbestos fibers.

Ken was short, but broad with balding brown hair and what appeared to be a slightly bigger head for his size. He wore glasses when he was reading or doing a telemedicine consult. He was well-liked by the house staff and was approachable due to his informal nature, the fact that he liked to jest, and that he always seemed to have a smile on his face. I thought of him as a maverick because he always had a unique, but appropriate, method and perspective. He walked expeditiously! Perhaps that was why sitting in stand-still traffic so frustrating for him.

It is clear that Dr. Bird's idea which I had initially thought was "stupid" had lit a spark in me that grew over time. Dr. Bird lit the flame on the torch that I would eventually carry beyond Massachusetts General Hospital.

It is hard for me to accept when people call me the Father of Telemedicine because, to me, that title should go to my professor, Dr. Kenneth Bird. Without Dr. Bird, where would telemedicine be? Would it exist? Maybe, but it certainly wouldn't have come about when it did. Dr. Bird birthed the idea during his sweaty drive under the Sumner

Tunnel in the summer of 1967, and inspired by his passion and quirks of fate, I would eventually adopt and raise it.

Who is the Father of Telemedicine? My co-author Michael Gorton and I constantly debate the issue.

From Michael Gorton: Jefferson and Adams did not invent democracy, but through their efforts, it became viable. Elon Musk did not invent the electric car, but he found a way to bring it into the mainstream. Nelson Mandela, an orphan, who was raised by an adopted father, changed the face of South Africa. We can stipulate that Jay Sanders did not create the idea of telemedicine, but as you will see in this book, he slogged through decades of resistance carrying the torch. Dr. Bird is the idea creator, but Sanders is the father. He adopted that child, and through decades of persistence, raised it like his own. It was Jay Sanders, who like Johnny Appleseed, visited medical schools over the years, planting the seeds that would ultimately blossom. In a later chapter, we will trace the genealogy of the seed Dr. Sanders planted that grew into Teladoc.

Coral Springs, FL

Halfway through my chief residency, the Chairman of the Department of Medicine, Dr. Alex Leaf approached me and requested I stay once my residency was complete. I was elated by his offer, but before I told him yes, I wanted to know if he had an interest in implementing an idea I had percolating in my mind. In the role of Chief Resident, I had the opportunity to go with all the attendings as they were rounding with the house staff. What struck me was that, when the attending was to be teaching the house staff about the patient's condition, they would be teaching through the lens of their specific specialty area. For example, if a patient came in with a diabetic foot ulcer due to neuropathy, the cardiologist attending would spend their time providing an excellent discussion of the pathophysiology and treatment of diabetic cardiomyopathy to the house staff, but not the condition for which the patient had been admitted, which was the diabetic neuropathy which had led to the foot ulcer. It seemed to me that an important piece was missing in our medical puzzle. As we were discussing my potential future at MGH, I took this time with Dr. Leaf to share an idea that I had for a new type of specialty practice.

"Dr. Leaf," I said, "I am humbled by your offer, but would like to express another need that the MGH has. You need a Division of General Medicine whose faculty is made up of specialty teachers who can discuss and teach on about 85% of the issues that arrive at the doorstep of this facility on a weekly basis. I want to help you build that."

Dr. Leaf was not interested, though he did reiterate his desire for me to stay, so I told him I wanted to take some more time to consider his offer. While I was thinking about it, I got a call from Dr. Bill Harrington, the well-known hematologist from Washington University who had recently identified the cause of idiopathic thrombocytopenic purpura (ITP) and had just been made the new Chairman of the Department of Medicine in Miami.

"Jay," he said, "I want you to be the Head of the House Staff program at the University of Miami's Jackson Memorial Hospital and become Assistant Chief of Medicine."

Now, I should admit that during those years many of my colleagues would have said I was crazy to turn down a faculty position at the MGH for a position at the University of Miami. However, given the sunny skies in Miami and the opportunity, I was thrilled by his offer, but I had to know if he would entertain my idea to create a Division of General Medicine with specialty teachers. Like Dr. Leaf, he said he didn't really understand what that was because, before then, there was no such thing as a Division of General Medicine. Yet, he told me that if I wanted to build that in addition to being the Head of the medical house staff program and Assistant Chief of Medicine, I could.

It also should be noted that Dr. Harrington offered me an annual salary of $25,000. At the time, that was such a large amount of money that I was embarrassed to tell people. It was almost more than the Chairman of the Department of Medicine at the Mass General was making at the time!

Motivated by an escape path from the infamous Boston traffic, the salary, the weather and, most importantly, the delusion that I could get the same good pizza in Miami (I couldn't), I packed up my family and we moved to Florida in the last week of December 1969. On January 1, 1970, I started the first Division of General Medicine in the country at the University of Miami. Today, there is a Division of General Medicine in every Department of Medicine in the country, so if I am to be identified as the "Father" of anything, it should be the "Division of General Medicine."

Once I got to Miami, life was crazy. I was attending on the wards for 11 of 12 months; I expanded the intensive care unit at Jackson Memorial Hospital and made morning and evening rounds in the ICU most of that first year. I took morning reports every day; I was starting and recruiting excellent teachers for the new Division of General Medicine, and along with my wife (who was a radiology resident at the time) I was learning how to be a parent to my young sons!

On top of that, the Dean of the University of Miami School of Medicine, Dr. Emanuel Papper, was having discussions with Mr. Tom Murrin, the president of one of the five major divisions of Westinghouse Electric, regarding a brand-new community development that would encompass "The Home of the Future," in Coral Springs, Florida. The project needed medical providers, and the dean was asking for my help getting something set up for them.

I suggested that we have primary care providers in Coral Springs but use Dr. Ken Bird's telemedicine system to communicate with the University of Miami for any specialty care needs. An infectious disease fellow, Dr. Joel Sachs, and my then Chief Resident, Dr. Chuck Wilhelm, said they would love to live in Coral Springs, and put money down on homes to be built. Westinghouse had agreed to pay for all the faculty salaries, would build and pay for a primary care clinic to be built on Sample Road and would pay for equipping it along with all the necessary telemedicine equipment.

At the last minute, Manny Papper reminded Tom Murrin that he would have to also pay the university overhead—which was about 40-50% at the time. Tom Murrin looked at Manny Papper like he was out of his mind. After that, everything fell apart. There would be no delivery of specialty care to Coral Springs via telemedicine. The first telemedicine initiative to a rural community in the early 1970s would not happen.

While discussions were taking place, and before everything fell apart, there was only one house at the Coral Springs development. It was the home of the future, called Electra 69. Remember, that was the summer that Neil, Buzz and Mike went to the Moon on Apollo XI. The future was here, and most everyone was embracing it. The Electra 69 was outfitted with all the shiny, new, cutting-edge Westinghouse Electric gadgets and was built by Westinghouse Electric with Mr. Joe Taravella, the developer. People would take tours of this and two other similar houses that were later built, ogling over the then state-of-the-art security cameras, the intercom system, the outdoor heating lamps, and portable his and hers panic buttons. Today, the Electra homes in Coral Springs have lost their shine and intrigue. What once was considered innovative is now an outdated artifact from a historic era.

Would that be the fate of telemedicine? Would it be presented with all the same excitement and enthusiasm as these futuristic homes only to quickly lose its relevance and become a thing of the past? Or would it stand the test of time?

CHAPTER 2

Jay H. Sanders, MD, FACP

Innovation in the Prisons

If I had asked the people what they wanted,
they would have said "a faster horse."
— Henry Ford

The RANN Initiative

As the 1960s ended, humanity saw the first moon landing on July 20, 1969, which was followed by five additional manned moon landings. Apollo 17, the final manned moon landing, occurred on December 19, 1972. The nation also watched the Watergate hearings on live TV. The (birth control) Pill and Roe v. Wade strengthened the Women's Liberation movement. The Vietnam War continued, as antiwar sentiment spread across the country.

The Beatles: John, Paul, George and Ringo, recorded their last album while the Eagles, Allman Brothers and Tom Petty rose to fame. A vast array of music was emerging, from soul to disco to punk. It was loud, experimental, and protest songs continued to be popular. Marvin Gaye's "What's Going On," and Crosby, Stills, Nash and Young's "Ohio," seem to elaborate well on the attitudes, protests, and riots of those tumultuous times.

The activist attitudes of those times were mirrored in prisons as well. On September 9, 1971, a riot broke out at the Attica Correctional Facility (prison) in New York, when prisoners on their way to breakfast took control of the prison, holding 39 guards hostage. Attica was notorious for having harsh living conditions. The prisoners were overcrowded, seldom allowed to shower, their letters and correspondence were censored, and they were allotted a mere one roll of toilet-paper per month. For those prisoners, proper healthcare was virtually non-existent. The inmates taking control of the prison that day sparked an outcry for change. That outcry was heard nationwide.

In the 1970s, healthcare for incarcerated individuals nationwide was neglectful at best. Overcrowding was not uncommon due to rising rates of imprisonment, and it was incredibly difficult to get doctors to work at correctional facilities. In addition, requests by inmates to be seen by a doctor were often met with skepticism by the prison guards. Often, prisoners could not get the care they needed at the prison, and, therefore, transport to the local hospital became necessary. For the high security facilities, transportation was risky…and expensive! Most state institutions required two correctional officers to oversee prisoner transport and visits to the hospital. In the federal system, depending on how dangerous the prisoner was determined to be, there could be as many as five correctional officers that would go with a single inmate!

During the time when I was at the University of Miami, and the Miami Dolphins were putting together the only perfect season in NFL history, the National Science

Foundation (NSF) had started a program called Research Applied to National Needs (RANN). In parallel, a similar initiative was started by the Department of Health and Human Services, then called Health Education and Welfare (HEW). They had set up these initiatives in response to a white paper published by the Institute of Electrical and Electronics Engineers, otherwise known as I Triple E, stating that telecommunications could have a dramatic effect in reducing the paucity of specialty care in rural areas.

I had all the equipment from the Coral Springs project collecting dust, so I was glad when the NSF asked me to apply for their program. Initially, I thought I would be bringing specialty care to rural communities via telemedicine, but the NSF had a different objective when they had asked me to apply. They wanted me to bring telemedicine technology to the correctional facility in Dade County, Florida. Wanting to ensure that this was a collective partnership, we applied as a triumvirate comprised of the county, the university, and a corporate entity, which were the Dade County Commissioner, Jackson Memorial Hospital (the teaching hospital for the University of Miami), and Westinghouse Electric respectively. The grant would enable us to test telemedicine technology at three facilities in the area: the main jail, the men's stockade, and the women's detention center.

I had long since become an advocate for the value of nurses and nurse practitioners, and as such, I was very interested in utilizing the capability of nurse practitioners in this project. There was just one small problem: there were no nurse practitioners in the state of Florida at that time! My colleagues were somewhat resistant to the idea that a nurse practitioner could do something as sophisticated as being the sole person caring for the patient. I, on the other hand, was of the mindset that I could not have made it through my residency and rounds without the nurses. When I became a first-year resident, I remember hugging the head nurse and telling her how much I appreciated her help during my internship. With that said, I wanted to return the favor by helping nurses realize their potential by becoming nurse practitioners.

I presented my idea to the dean of the School of Nursing at the University of Miami, and she was very receptive. We created an extremely accelerated six-month nurse practitioner program, then asked six incredible nurses from the Jackson Memorial Hospital Emergency Department if they would be interested. As I remember, those six ED nurses plus the Dean and Associate Dean of the School of Nursing became the first eight nurse practitioners in the state of Florida. This, much to the dismay of many of my fellow physicians licensed and practicing in the state. They would be our experimental group, on-site at the correctional facilities, connected via telemedicine with a team of physicians at Jackson Memorial Hospital.

For the three-year study for the NSF, we evaluated four parameters:

1. The cost of care (including the technology)
2. The quality of care
3. The psychological impact (how did the doctors nurses, and inmates feel about care given at a distance?) and
4. The technology (how well did it function?)
   We sent the four-volume report to the NSF in early 1976 showing the obvious benefit of nurse practitioners using telemedicine in prisons.

At the same time, there were about six to eight other programs funded by the NSF and HEW for telemedicine. One of those fascinating programs was a study done by Dr. Sam Pool, who worked for NASA, with HEW. In preparation for working laboratories in space, including the International Space Station (ISS), NASA was brainstorming ways of providing medical care to the astronauts who would be living on the ISS. Dr. Pool wanted to demonstrate that satellite transmission could be used for the communication network for a telemedicine initiative.

A sidebar that is worth mentioning is that most of us were using microwave transmission for our telemedicine systems, which is incredibly susceptible to lightning. Florida, the Sunshine State, is also known for having the highest number of lightning bolts per year in the United States. The State sees an average of 3,500 lightning strikes touch the ground *each day*. It is also the highest in lightning related fatalities nationwide. Dade County specifically was widely hit by lightning, so it was constantly disrupting our system! If we could have used satellite transmission then, we obviously could have avoided that issue.

Dr. Pool's two objectives were to evaluate the use of satellite transmission of telemedicine services to the projected Space Station as well as here on Earth to the Papago Reservation in Arizona. Unfortunately, Dr. Pool's goal of delivering telemedicine to native Americans failed as a result of an anemic budget coupled with cultural barriers that made it challenging to deliver telehealth to the Native American population. However, his study was extremely successful in proving that satellite to ground transmission could provide effective interactive capabilities.

During this same time, my professor Dr. Ken Bird, also received a grant to continue his work at the Massachusetts General. An additional project was being implemented by an anesthesiology department chairman who was using the technology in various operating rooms in his network to watch the newer anesthesiologists do their work.

Many of these programs, including ours, demonstrated that telemedicine was an incredibly effective means of delivering healthcare. My correctional care project demonstrated not only the viability of telemedicine, but perhaps more importantly, that an on-site doctor could be supplanted by nurse practitioners utilizing telemedicine. The end result was less transportation required, more immediate care, and decreased costs and security requirements for patient inmate health care needs.

We produced a four-volume report that planted the seeds which we had hoped would ultimately spark the telemedicine revolution. Interestingly, in the near term, the report was reviewed by the governments of Iran and the Philippines and in 1976, I was invited to consult with them to address some of the issues they were facing in providing adequate healthcare to their people.

In the longer term, our success with the innovative use of telecommunications to address the health care needs of inmates would lead to the adoption of this form of medical care access in some of the larger correctional care programs across the country. Little did we realize that this innovation in delivery and access would experience pointless opposition from the very bodies that should have embraced it. Our Jackson Memorial program and those that followed, sat under the protective umbrella of the Federal and State governments, and were not subject to the scrutiny of the State Boards, the AMA, the DEA, the Nursing Boards, and some of the other entities that would later whole-heartedly resist the inevitable Telemedicine and Digital Care Revolution.

Louie Wainwright and Telemedicine for Florida's Department of Corrections

Once the results came out from our NSF grant looking at the application of telemedicine for the three correctional care facilities in Florida as well as the effective utilization of nurse practitioners in this setting, we got a call from the then Secretary of the Department of Corrections for the state of Florida, Louie Wainwright, asking if we could start an experimental program for the state of Florida. Louie was thought of as a forward thinker in terms of the rights of inmates. He was kind, humble, unpretentious, and passionate about human rights. He was a well-liked and respected man in his field.

Louie specifically wanted the use of telemedicine for their intake facilities in northern Florida. In those days, they would process the inmates going on to different prisons at a single intake facility, where several inmates would be placed in the same cell. They were particularly interested in teleradiology, so that chest X-rays could be evaluated more quickly to ensure that tuberculosis was not communicated from one inmate to the many others confined to the same cell. The application of telemedicine in correctional care, as taught to me by Louie Wainwright, was an obvious choice, not simply because of tuberculosis and overcrowded cells. Prisons are usually in rural areas because most people don't like to have them near the cities and suburbs where they live and work.

It can also benefit rural communities by bringing jobs in the form of correctional officers who often live and spend their money in that community. However, the disadvantage of prisons being in rural areas is that, when an inmate gets sick, they must be transferred a considerable distance to get effective medical care. As mentioned previously, this also meant that many times at least two correctional officers (and in the Federal system depending on the nature of the inmate, as many as five correctional officers) would have to accompany the inmate to the hospital to ensure safety. This was costly, especially because in most situations, the guard(s) accompanying the inmate were on overtime status because the warden did not want to diminish their security capability in the correctional facility. And as is obvious, to transport an inmate was a much riskier process than it would be to bring a doctor in virtually via telemedicine, which is what made it the obvious choice for correctional care.

Based on this, the first commercial correctional healthcare telemedicine program was introduced in the state of Florida. This laid the roots for the subsequent program in the state with the largest prison system in the United States: Texas. In addition, shortly after the program was up and running in Florida, and its subsequent iteration in Texas, the idea was adopted by many private companies who would be contracted out by prisons to deliver healthcare. Today, telemedicine is widely used in correctional care facilities.

CHAPTER 3

Jay H. Sanders, MD, FACP

The Naïve Consultant

Education is the most powerful weapon,
Which you can use to change the world
— Nelson Mandela

I find it amazing how the seeds of an idea can be scattered worldwide by technology—even that which we possessed in the 70s. As we posted results on our projects, information was carried around the world, and interested parties reached out. In my case, I had the opportunity to meet leaders of countries, to teach them about telemedicine, and change the way their governments contributed to the citizens' health. I use the word opportunity because I went into those environments with the wrong priority. What happened instead, was I learned something truly valuable.

The Shah of Iran

Shah Mohammad Reza Pahlavi was the final ruler to hold that role before the Iranian Revolution in 1979. Shah Mohammad had a vision for a "Great Civilization," as he called it, which would be a literate, educated, rich, and more democratic populace. He also had a fascination with all the latest technological advances. The Shah had a vision for his "Great Civilization," along with an affinity for gadgets.

The combination of these two interests must have played into his invitation for me to visit Iran in August 1976. Both the Shah and I held hopes of bringing telemedicine to his country.

Michael's note:

I had a personal connection to the "Great Civilization" while attending engineering school at the University of Texas. The Shah was willing to pay the expenses for any citizen willing to attend engineering school in the US. Several of my fellow engineering students in 1977 and 1978 were Iranians who I studied with and befriended. I quickly learned that not only were their academic expenses covered, but they all had nice cars, ample expense accounts, and lived in the nicer apartments. Being an engineering student was a well-paid job for those young Persians, whose primary objective was to bring technology back to their home country.

Sadly, many of them did not appreciate the value. As the revolution lit up, many of them supported it in the beginning, then later changed that stance, as they were declared enemies of the state.

Jay H. Sanders, MD

Someone in the Iranian government read one of my reports or articles and became fascinated by the prospect. With this, I accepted a personal invitation from the Shah to assess, educate, and implement. Upon arrival, I found an incredibly enthusiastic Shah, enamored with all manner of gadgets, but he particularly adored the US Air Force F-86 Sabrejet. And no wonder—the F-86 was the first swept wing trans sonic fighter. As I recall, the majority of his entire military air force was made up of US Sabrejets with Iranian insignias. Interestingly, the engine mechanics for his jets were predominantly Israeli, and in return for their service, the Shah would provide Israel with oil. Given the conflict that now exists between Israel and Iran, it is hard to imagine the two countries in collaboration, much less the working friendship in existence at that time.

The Shah wanted to bring telemedicine to Iran for all the right reasons. Healthcare existed mostly in Tehran, the capital, and some other major cities, such as Shiraz, where there was the Pahlavi Medical School, named after the royal family. The Shah had a dream of bringing healthcare to the outlying communities. Based on everything I had seen while I was there, however, I believed then that their needs were much more basic. I had never been exposed to the kind of poverty I saw on my visit to Iran. People were living in mud huts, often with the livestock residing with them. I was also struck by the irony that there were people working diligently to sweep the streets of Tehran, but the sewage was flowing in open-air gutters along those same clean streets.

In the mid-1970s, the country was an interesting amalgamation of high tech and third world living conditions, woven together by a dictatorial regime that ruled with an iron fist. In spite of this, there were sparks of good. My visit provided a window where I could see the potential, engulfed in difficulties. I was there, at the behest of the Shah, who wanted to give this innovative concept of tele-medicine to people who had practically no modern care.

Still, my naivete prevailed.

When asked by the Shah what I thought, I informed him that I believed there was a much higher priority than telemedicine in improving healthcare in his country and his people. I advised him that the best first step, in my opinion, should be to fix sanitation and food issues before spending his money on telemedicine.

For years, I questioned my personal recommendation. I often wonder what would have happened if I had just said, "Yes! Let's do this!" In the US, at the time, the people in power were largely opposed to the idea of telemedi-cine. The State Boards said that a physician should not be allowed to treat a patient she has never touched. They said doctors should not be allowed to practice in states where they are not licensed. And while they were enforcing those "doctrines," the Shah was willing to fund and support the first nationwide telemedicine program in the world.

I left Iran with little more than an idealistic memory. What might have been? We will never know. Within a few years, the Shah would be diagnosed with cancer, and the regime would fall to Ayatollah Khomeini. For all its good and bad, the collaborative friendship between Iran and Israel and the United States would dissolve into tension.

Interestingly, within weeks of my refusal to help build a telemedicine program in Iran, I was invited to the Pacific Island nation of the Philippines.

Ferdinand and Imelda

In September1976, when I had received my invitation from President Ferdinand Marcos, and his wife Imelda, the Philippines was still a newborn independent republic. The Pacific Island country had been granted independence from the United States on July 4, 1946. In his first presidential term from 1965 to1969, Ferdinand Marcos was admired by his country as a decorated war hero. Imelda was known as the "Steel Butterfly," due to her political drive along with her always-glamorous attire. His ambition and strength, coupled with her allure, made them a political power couple in the Philippines. Because of a prosperous and successful first term and the Marcos' popularity, Ferdinand Marcos was the first president in the Philippines to be re-elected for a second term.

Shortly into Marcos' second term, however, things began to get rocky. Social unrest led Marcos to declare martial law in 1972. Those who opposed Marcos were silenced. The media was censored. The constitution was ratified. In 1975, President Marcos made Imelda the governor of Metro Manila, thus usurping the person who had been elected governor! Marcos became known over the course of his 20-year rule over the Philippines as an authoritarian dictator.

Interestingly, less than a year prior to my visit, one of the most famous boxing matches of all time took place in Manila. The match was between Joe Frazier and Muhammad Ali and was dubbed the Thrilla in Manila. Ali won that match.

Michael's note:

Lovers of history may recall that it was the Philippines where Ferdinand Magellan met his end in April 1521. Magellan was killed by a poison arrow in a skirmish called the Battle of Mactan. His historic circumnavigation of the globe was finally completed by Juan Sebastian de Elcano in September 1522.

In the early days of World War II, while under assault by Japanese forces, General Douglas MacArthur fled the Philippines with the famous words: "I shall return." Near the end of the war in October 1944, MacArthur fulfilled that promise when he re-took the island of Leyte.

My own personal connection to the Philippines was in the early 70s when I lived on the Island of Luzon, in Angeles City. My father, an Air Force sergeant, was stationed at Clark Air Force Base. I was in the sixth grade. The PI, as we called it (Philippine Islands), was a constant adventure for a young intrepid kid. With the jungles, cobras, volcanoes, headhunters, cannibals, and gun battles, there was never a shortage of danger and excitement. Marcos was the president and was still loved and admired. Much of the population lived in thatched nipa huts, elevated above the ground by piers, constructed mostly of bamboo. Those huts typically lacked electricity and running water. Healthcare was a luxury afforded to a small fraction of the populace.

Jay H. Sanders, MD, FACP

Like with the Shah, I received a personal invitation to visit President and Mrs. Marcos to evaluate bringing telemedicine to the PI. This visit occurred in the beginning of September 1976. Prior to my visit, I was advised that the country was under martial law. When I got to the airport, I was met by government officials, and suddenly two women approached and started measuring me! My first thought was, "Oh my God! They are measuring me for a coffin—just in case!" Actually, these women were seamstresses and what they were doing was measuring me to be fitted for my own barong Tagalog, the ornate, embroidered national shirt of the Philippines! I would be having several dinners at the presidential palace over the course of my stay, and they wanted me to be properly outfitted. Incidentally, I have kept and treasure those barongs to this day.

The Philippines is made up of an archipelago of over 7,000 islands, the major one being Luzon, where Manila, the capital, is situated. In Metro Manila, there were specialty medical institutes, including a cardiology institute. Appropriately, Mrs. Marcos wanted to use telemedicine to bring the expertise of cardiologists and other specialists in Metro

Manila to the archipelago islands to improve the health of the people.

As I toured this magnificent panoramic country, once again I was struck by the lack of sanitation, food, and access to primary care outside of Metro Manila. The outlying communities and islands were still inhabited heavily by indigenous people living in primitive conditions.

My naivete led me to advise President and Mrs. Marcos, just as I had advised the Shah, that the priority should not be telemedicine, but to first solve sanitation and food issues. Also, like my visit with the Shah, it was the side aspects of my trip that were most fascinating. I had the privilege of attending a few dinners with Ferdinand and Imelda while I was there, and I was impressed with President Marcos' gift for extemporaneous speeches!

Near the end of my week there, President Marcos asked if I would like to go to the Island of Corregidor to see some movies about the Second World War that had never been shown in the movie theaters in the United States. As a kid, I frequented the movie theater. In those days, you would see two movies, a news segment by Pathé News, and a cartoon! On Saturdays, my parents would send me off with a sack lunch and I would spend my day there, often seeing pictures about the War. So, when President Marcos asked me to go with him to the movies, I eagerly agreed!

We departed from Manila Bay aboard President Marcos' personal ship, flanked by a search and destroy vessel and a hospital vessel. President Marcos had also invited a woman who was the president of Chiquita Banana at the time. The four of us went to Corregidor, saw these movies, and on our way back, we had a meal on the deck. We were having a lovely time!

I remember that President Marcos was sitting across from me, the President of Chiquita Banana was on my left and Imelda was on my right. Approximately half-way through our dinner, an aide walked up to President Marcos and whispered something in his ear. Immediately, his facial expression changed.

"Dr. Sanders," he said gravely, "you will have to excuse me. I have just been informed that Chairman Mao has died."

My reaction was joy, but thankfully, I did not celebrate.

Upon hearing this news, Imelda Marcos grabbed my arm and exclaimed, "Oh! How terrible!"

Here I was, a young, naïve American who yet had much to learn about the way the world works, wondering why our ally, the Philippines, was so troubled that the leader of communist China had died!

"Why are you so upset?" I asked Mrs. Marcos, genuinely curious.

"You do not know Chairman Mao like we do!" Imelda explained, "Oh, he was a wonderful man, a leader of his country, a poet, and a philosopher. We had many state visits together."

Imelda promised me that when I got home, she would send me pictures from one of their state visits. I'm not sure whether I still have those pictures, but I remember that, in one picture, Chairman Mao wore a cap and a gray uniform and stood between President and Mrs. Marcos with his arms around them.

In retrospect, I believed that I had valuable information to teach the leaders of Iran and the Philippines. I had been invited to these two countries as a consultant, but the truth is, I became the student! These two experiences, far from home, were indispensable lessons in my education about how the world works, how useful telemedicine could be across the globe. Yet, we were so far from seeing that realized!

Unlike Magellan, the idea of telemedicine did not die in the PI. More like MacArthur, I learned a valuable lesson that would ultimately drive my interest in bringing remote care to the US and to the world.

The Yunnan Province

The Yunnan Province in China is a land of diversity. The terrain varies from rice-terraces to snow-capped mountains to mountain gorges. The province is also ethnically diverse, being home to about half of the ethnic minority groups in China. I had the privilege of visiting this place in south-western China in the late 90s, twenty years after my visits to Iran and the Philippines. The objective, however, was similar: to evaluate whether telemedicine would be appropriate for the area.

I was invited to southwestern China by SunPa, a

government tax supported computer company. At the time, they were only a small computer company, but they were interested in starting a telemedicine program, so they invited me to stay for a week. I arrived in Hong Kong then flew from there via China Airways to Yunnan Province. They put me up in a hotel in the capital city of Kunming, and I remember waking up there on the first morning and looking out the window to see what must have been half the city doing Tai Chi around the lake! It was beautiful and enchanting to watch.

What an experience it was to visit this part of China! The cuisine, mirroring the landscape and the people, is an amalgam of the variety of cultures living in the province. "Crossing the bridge noodles," wild mushrooms made in a hot pot of flavorful broth, pineapple rice, and roast duck are among the most popular traditional foods I may have eaten in my time there. I remember that the food was incredible!

I visited rural communities of million-plus people, two 750-bed hospitals, and talked to many physicians there. It seemed to me that they were simply not up to date with what we were doing in the United States. I was struck by the thought, just as I had been in Iran and the Philippines, that this was not the best first step. Additionally, I met with the CEO of SunPa and two of his brothers, who were vice presidents of the company. They expressed to me their hope to start up a telemedicine program, their specific interest being in teleradiology. Looking back, I believe this would have been simple to implement. At the time, however, I was skeptical, naïve, or both.

At the end of the week, I attended a state dinner hosted by the provincial governor. I remember the governor walking over to me and asking me with a smile and a look of pride, "Well, Dr. Sanders, what do you think about our idea of bringing telemedicine to the outlying communities?"

"It's a wonderful idea," I said, "but there are some more basic steps I feel you should make. I don't think telemedicine should be your first step."

I will never forget how she responded to me.

"I know this is not the best first step, but it is a step, and it will act like a magnet and cause all the other necessary steps to happen."

She was absolutely correct, and just as in Iran and the Philippines years before, I failed to realize that sometimes the quickest and most effective way to solve a social problem may not be a step-by-step approach. Flying home from that visit, I thought to myself that I had gone there as a consultant, and I was flying back as a student. It was one of the great lessons of my life.

UAE

In late 1988 or 1989, I received a call from Dr. Raymond Levey, a transplant surgeon and friend, formerly with Boston Children's Hospital. Ray was a consultant to the UAE, specifically Abu Dhabi, and he was calling to ask if I would go with him to Abu Dhabi to talk with them about the application of telemedicine. Of course, I accepted and went along with him. The Minister of Health was very interested in deploying telehealth in the UAE for a specific practical reason, and it had the potential to be extremely successful because he already had the communication infrastructure in place! A little-known fact about the UAE was that they had an exceptional communication infrastructure. They had cell phones basically before anyone else in the Middle East.

The UAE government paid for all the medical expenses of its citizens, but unfortunately, it was difficult to find medical expertise in the UAE. So, what did the citizens do? They went abroad, and the government was paying for everything—from plane tickets to hotel and meals, to their medical visits. Upon investigation the Minister of Health had made an interesting discovery. Many of the citizens who were traveling abroad for a second opinion were missing their first appointments and having to reschedule! At first this was puzzling. Why travel all the way from the UAE to London, NYC, Rochester in Minnesota, or Boston only to miss your appointment?

The question of why so many people truly wanted to go abroad was answered simply and quite comically: they wanted to go abroad to shop! Many of them would have minor dermatologic problems and would schedule an appointment with a dermatologist at, for example, the Mayo Clinic in Rochester, Minnesota, to go shopping at the Mall of America! Huge amounts of money were being spent by the UAE government so that people could go on vacations and shopping sprees.

What Ray Levey suggested was that a hospital of the future be built in Glasgow, Scotland. Professors from Mayo Clinic, Boston, and England were being paid very highly to drop their contracts, leave their schools, and fill the various specialty departments at this hospital in Glasgow. An enormous hospital was built, the doors were opened...and nobody came. Upon analysis of why, it was discovered that no one wanted to go to Glasgow because there was very little shopping there!

Not long after, the UAE's Health Minister was promoted to Oil Minister, and all interest in telemedicine dissipated. Perhaps it never would have worked anyway because it seemed what the people really wanted was to shop. Yet, the common thread weaving through all these stories is that, at the time, there was significant international interest in telemedicine—from Iran to the Philippines to China to the UAE. Meanwhile, most bureaucrats in the United States either were doing everything they could to choke it out of existence or worse yet, ignoring its ability to address access to healthcare for those who had been disenfranchised because of access, infrastructure and/or cost.

Norway

Steiner Pedersen was the head of the Ear, Nose and Throat Department at the University of Tromso in Tromso, Norway. He invited me to visit as a telemedicine consultant in the mid-90s. His impetus for telemedicine came from the fact that there were very few ENT specialists in the country of Norway. Typically, when a primary care physician would have an ENT problem arise, they would send them to Tromso. If you are unfamiliar with the geography of Norway, Tromso is nearly as far north as one can go in mainland Norway. It would likely require a flight to get from any of the other major cities, like Oslo, Bergen, or Stavanger to Tromso. Of course, because all medical expenses are covered by the Norwegian government, travel and stay would be paid for, but not entirely convenient.

During my stay in Norway, I was served an obscene amount of salmon. Allow me to be clear that I *love* salmon! However, I was served salmon at breakfast, lunch, and dinner. There was salmon mousse, smoked salmon, salmon eggs, and I swear, there may have even been a salmon dessert! I was entirely salmon-ed out before the end of my trip, so I resolved to go in search of a non-salmon meal. I sat down at a restaurant, ordered a burger, and soon came to find out that it was a reindeer burger! The food I have enjoyed in the many countries telemedicine has taken me has always been an interesting and enlightening part of the experience!

Dr. Pedersen was one of the early pioneers in the use of telemedicine by utilizing the technology to examine patients in their primary care offices without the need for the patient to travel. What needs to be emphasized in all the years that I have been doing telemedicine is that besides bringing necessary care to the patient, it dramatically increases the continuing education of the physician!

Recall that most physicians are trained at major academic medical centers where they have access to every sub-specialty expertise.

Then, a physician might enter a rural healthcare setting where he or she is all by themselves and all that specialty expertise is no longer right there at their fingertips. Prior to telemedicine, it used to be that physician turnover in rural areas was alarmingly high, which would further contribute to the paucity of quality physicians in rural settings. However, telemedicine has helped solve this problem by bringing that continuing education directly to the rural setting, like it did in Norway and has in the US.

CHAPTER 4

Jay H. Sanders, MD, FACP

The U.S. Wakes Up

Whatever the mind of man can conceive and believe,
It can achieve
— Napoleon Hill

Georgia Leads the Way

D r. Francis Tedesco is known as the doctor who identified a gut bacterium called clostridium difficile,
which killed a lot of immunosuppressed people. He also
identified the antibiotic that would destroy it. The irony of
it is that C. difficile is caused by overuse of several antibiotics, but, there was one capable of killing it, and Dr. Tedesco
identified which one. In the early 1970s, I had recruited Fran
when he was a GI Fellow at Barnes Hospital at the University of Washington to be a member of the newly formed
and first Division of General Medicine at the University
of Miami. It was around that time that I received the NSF
telemedicine grant, and Fran saw firsthand the results
and capabilities of telemedicine. After about four years of
being in Miami, Fran left for the Medical College of Georgia to become head of their Division of Gastroenterology,
for which I had written him a letter of recommendation.
Eventually, Dr. Tedesco was promoted to President of the
Medical College of Georgia.

In October 1991, I received a call from Fran inviting me
to visit him at the Medical College of Georgia to discuss the

potential for utilizing telemedicine for the State of Georgia. The then governor of Georgia, Zell Miller, was interested in this subject because he had discussed with Dr. Tedesco what we had done in the early 1970s with the NSF grant. To my surprise, when I first met the governor, he introduced himself as the governor of two states.

Looking at him quizzically, I said, "Excuse me, Governor?"

"Yes, Jay," he said, "I am the governor of Atlanta and the governor of the rest of Georgia."

He explained to me that they had everything they needed from a healthcare delivery standpoint in Atlanta, but nowhere near enough in the rest of Georgia, which was predominantly rural. This was why Zell Miller was so interested in telemedicine. He also gave me a crash course in Economics 101, which I had not taken in medical school.

In Georgia, as well as in many rural states across the US, many of the hospitals in rural communities were closing because of a declining bed census. Because they didn't have the necessary level of expertise, patients were transferred to secondary and tertiary care facilities, so the small hospitals just didn't have enough patients. For example, when a patient was admitted to a rural hospital with a complex problem like a stroke, there were no neurologists, so the patient was immediately transferred to another hospital. In many cases, people knew themselves they couldn't receive the care they needed at the rural hospital, so they would go directly to a secondary or tertiary care facility.

From an economics standpoint, Zell Miller taught me that the closure of a rural hospital was detrimental to the community because, he said, that within a 3-5-year period the entire socioeconomic infrastructure of that community is destroyed because the hospital had been the major employer in town. For that reason, Zell Miller's interest in telemedicine was twofold: he hoped to both bring specialty healthcare to rural communities and to stabilize the economy of rural Georgia.

At that time, Verizon had not bought up all the smaller telecommunications companies yet, and Bell Atlantic was a major provider. The president of Bell South, which serviced Georgia, was a Mr. Carl Swearingen, who also was the head of a technology counsel which the governor had established. I do not remember the reason, but Bell Atlantic, Georgia had been fined for something, and there was this fund of $50 million that the governor of Georgia controlled. After talking with Carl Swearingen, he became very interested in helping to implement telemedicine by putting in the communication infrastructure and be able to use the funds that his company had been fined to accomplish the task!

So, I came up as a consultant to the Medical College of Georgia, and we created the first state-wide telemedicine network consisting of fifty-nine sites. There were three anchor tertiary care centers: one was Emory, one was the Medical College of Georgia, and the third was in Macon. We connected those to nine comprehensive community hospitals, which were secondary care facilities that had essentially all the necessary sub-specialties. Those, in turn, were networked to rural hospitals, several correctional facilities, a nursing home, a number of free-standing AHEC facilities, and, if memory serves me, one public school.

There was only one problem at the time that curtailed our ability to do a complete examination utilizing the system we put in place. Based on the feedback that we received from the primary care physicians in these rural hospitals, they wanted the ability for us to examine their patients besides simply having an audio-video capability. In essence, they were asking us to corroborate the findings they noted when examining the patient. Electronic devices for looking into the ear, nose, throat and the eyes of the patient over telemedicine did not yet exist. We even had requests for our GI specialist to be able to watch an internist who had taught himself how to do gastroscopy. This inspired our bioengineering division at the Medical College of Georgia to build tiny cameras that could be attached to the ends of the scoping devices. Those became the first peripheral diagnostic devices for telemedicine! If I recall correctly, we subsequently ended up demonstrating how we did this to some commercial specialty device companies.

After we had completed this 59-site, inter-connected telemedicine system, a neurologist, for example, could now be connected to a patient who had just come into the ER at a small hospital in rural Georgia and quickly identify what was going on—whether it was a bleed or a thrombus. Where this became life-saving and beneficial was that a thrombolytic agent now could be given within the correct time frame that would dissolve the clot, leading to revascularization of the infarcted area. Now a patient who previously would have been paralyzed, could walk out of the hospital within a few days with no deficit. This system was saving lives!

The Exam Room is Where the Patient Lives, Not Where the Doctor Works

Something that became apparent within the first couple of months of implementing Georgia's telemedicine system is that we began to see some so called "revolving door patients", meaning they would be discharged, and within a short time later be re-admitted to the hospital. The classic example was the patient with asthma, particularly in the winter months. They would come into the ER in extremis, would have to be intubated, and then sent off to the intensive care unit, where they would be stabilized, and eventually sent home. Their pulmonary function studies would be almost normal on discharge, but then within a two- or three-week period, they would be back in the emergency room.

I thought, Wait a minute! What is going on here? We must be missing something!

Working with the bioengineering division of Georgia Tech, where I was a senior research faculty member, as well as having been appointed Professor of Medicine and Surgery at the Medical College of Georgia, we applied for a grant to the federal government to do something that had not been done before: to bring telemedicine into the home and basically the only technology that existed in the early 90s was the home television. I figured if I could just do follow-up examinations of the patient in their home, I might be able to figure out what was causing them to be re-admitted so quickly, and potentially prevent their subsequent ER admissions!

This was 1993, so remember that the internet was not yet in homes and there was no smart phone. Yet, we postulated that if we could connect to the patient utilizing their TV, we could achieve the capability of examining them in their home. Working with Georgia Tech, we put in a grant request to the Federal Government and received about a million dollars to see if we could do it. When we received the grant, we also received interest in the project from Colonel Fred Goeringer who headed the Medical Advanced Technology Management Office (MATMO), as it was called at the time, (now TATRC—Telemedicine Advanced Technology research Center) at Fort Detrick, Maryland. He was particularly interested in teleradiology, but when he heard what we were doing, he came down to visit. He added some funds, but also asked that we involve Fort Gordon in Augusta, Georgia, which is the signaling center for the DOD.

We then received a call from the local cable company, Jones Intercable, who told me they could help us make the

TV two-way-interactive, and they wanted to do it on their own dime!

"Why would you do this?!" I asked them.

"Think about it, Jay! If your system works, we will have a medical health channel and in the same way we charge the people a monthly fee for the movie channel, we will charge them a monthly fee for the medical channel! So, we are happy to spend our money to do this."

They did say there would be one small problem with the technology. We, of course, did not have fiber optics back then, we just had coaxial cable, and while they could make the system two-way interactive, everyone who was put on the system would be on a party line. This meant that if there were two emergencies or people needing care at the same time, we could only help one. However, this was an experiment, so I said I wanted to go forward with it and see what we could do.

We would call the system the "Electronic House Call." We identified about twenty of our "revolving door" patients, and I will never forget the first patient we saw over the system when it was complete in 1995. She was a patient with severe asthma who was sitting in a big, fluffy chair with a cat on her lap and her spouse smoking a cigarette in the doorway. All these things are major red flags for patients with asthma! I would never have observed this scene had the patient come into the office. This single event made me realize that the best exam room is where the patient lives, not where the doctor works!

You can catch so many problems in the patient's home environment that you would never see or even know existed at the hospital or doctor's office. Another example of this would be an elderly patient who has a step down from the living room to the kitchen or low-lighting going up the stairs, which are all fall-hazards or the patient who sleeps in one position for too long, which can cause bed sores, or forgets they left the stove on. That first telemedicine house-call fundamentally changed everything I had previously thought about where patient care should occur, and I have been focusing on the home ever since then. In many respects, this Electronic House Call of 1995 presaged what we see today in terms of remote patient monitoring and the "hospital-at-home" movement.

To Arizona, California, and Beyond

Shortly after telemedicine was initiated in the state of Georgia, I received a call from Dr. Ron Weinstein from the University of Arizona asking if he could come with a legislative delegation to see our system. Why Ron Weinstein? Well, he had been a resident in the Department of Pathology at Massachusetts General Hospital and participated in Ken Bird's telemedicine program as I had. Ron clearly knew the potential, therefore, that telemedicine could mean for his State of Arizona. He simply needed to convince the legislature to provide the necessary funding. Because of that visit, the State of Arizona now has committed funding on a yearly basis for the maintenance and expansion of Ron's program, which is one of the premier statewide programs in the USA.

Following Arizona, representatives from UC Davis in California came to evaluate the system, and that led to the initiation of their program as well, and became the pattern of telemedicine integration into all the existing statewide programs today. I do not think it would be an overstatement to indicate that if it were not for Dr. Fran Tedesco and then Governor Zell Miller's initiative to bring healthcare to rural Georgia via telemedicine in the early 1990s, this country would not have been as well prepared to address the needs of the healthcare community during the COVID Pandemic.

Telemedicine for Texas' Department of Corrections

In the mid-1990s, the Texas legislature passed a bill that mandated care be delivered to inmates within 24 hours. In the beginning, an attempt was made to deliver that care through traditional in-person delivery. I met with Oscar Boultinghouse at the University of Texas Medical (UTMB) branch in Galveston, bringing Dr. Boultinghouse and his team up to speed on our success in Georgia and other programs. At the time, I never would have predicted the sequence of events that would spin out of that meeting.

The UTMB correctional care team just happened to be located adjacent to the office of a NASA Space Systems Engineer and flight surgeon named G. Byron Brooks, an electrical engineer and medical doctor. Doctor Brooks had spent a short period of time as an operations officer at Internet Global handling audio and video data communications, a company started by my co-author, Michael Gorton.

By the late 1990s, I had been planting the seeds of telemedicine, never knowing which will grow. Doctor Boultinghouse had responsibility for the largest correctional care contract in the US, and that led to Dr. Brooks, who clearly had two of the essential ingredients—a working knowledge of telecom engineering and a medical degree. As fate would have it, Dr. Brooks added another ingredient that would be inserted later: his best friend was a serial entrepreneur.

A note from G. Byron Brooks, EE, MD

After the Texas legislature passed the bill requiring care to be delivered to inmates requesting medical care within 24-hours but prior to the application of telemedicine in prisons, physicians were putting themselves in harm's way to deliver in-person care. Physicians and healthcare providers visiting the prisons had experienced more than their share of violence, including one who had his throat slashed, another cornered by inmates, feces thrown at them, one was raped, and one killed.

Another issue was that inmates would often fake injuries or hurt themselves on a Friday afternoon and ask to go to the hospital just to get a weekend away from the prison. When you consider that at least two guards had to accompany the inmate and remain with them for the duration of their hospital stay, this got very expensive. The application of telemedicine to prisons would solve these problems!

In 1999, Dr. Boultinghouse and I agreed we would deliver primary care, in addition to specialty care, to the Texas Department of Criminal Justice (TDCJ) prisons. First, however, we would have to sell the system to the wardens and unit medical staff, and not every unit wanted us initially. Texas State Penitentiary at Huntsville and Carole S. Young Medical Facility were among the first few to give approval to proceed. Slowly but surely, it spread, and we were eventually delivering care in about 99% of the units across the state. As I recall, that was somewhere around eighty-thousand patients. That made us the largest telemedicine program in the world.

When we first got started, I remember seeing around four patients per day. Our efficiency and skills grew to the point where, on one record day, Dr. Boultinghouse and I saw more than 100 patients.

Our telemedicine setup consisted of a desktop computer and a remotely controlled camera, which we would put on a cart and wheel it up to the patient's cell, or place in the unit's medical exam room, as needed. The physician could see the patient, and the patient could also see the physician. With a remote-controlled camera, the physician could change angles or zoom in or out as needed. There was the option for the telemedicine doctor to use a special studio-like room that the UTMB group had set up with three large computer screens, a giant wooden desk, a remote control for the camera, and a big higher definition screen to observe the patient. With all that tech, often I would be handling patient consults from a much simpler setup in the convenience of my home or university office.

While our most significant advancement was building the largest telemedicine program to date, we created a few tech innovations for the service. To enable physicians to listen to the patient's heart-tones, I developed a stethoscope that had a microphone at the end of it. We had an ophthalmoscope and an otoscope that would send pictures back to our system, and we would have a nurse or technician on site with the patient who we could advise where we needed the stethoscope placed or where to hold the ophthalmoscope or otoscope.

As you might imagine, the images were rudimentary, so it was key for the physician to establish a rapport with the patient and draw them in so that they would trust the physician and *tell* him or her what was wrong with them. I would say that about 80% of the information that helped me treat the patient, I collected from the conversation that I had with them. As we all learned in medical school: if you listen to the patients, they will tell you what's wrong with them!

Since we were doing primary care, most of the patients we treated had minor issues like colds, diabetes, depression, headaches, and the flu. If there was an emergency like a stab wound, we would put them in an ambulance to be transferred to the hospital. I had some patients who had more serious communicable diseases like multi-drug resistant tuberculosis with AIDS or HIV or systemic uncontrolled herpes zoster, and I would review their records, talk to them, and check in on them. Sometimes I would make in-person visits, but complicated issues would typically be handed off to a specialist. Many of those patients ended up getting shipped off to Galveston, which had a prison hospital with specialist care, operating rooms, inmate expertise and more.

The Board of Medical Examiners was concerned about our foray into telemedicine. I think because of the UTMB and state of Texas connections, they did not actively try to shut us down. In fact, while they took a skeptical view, Dr. Boultinghouse and I both became recognized experts to some members of the Board. As another value-added twist, there were only about 12-15 pediatric psychiatrists in the state of Texas at that time. Using our telemedicine assets, I applied for and received a grant for $5 million to set up systems in various cities around the state to help deliver pediatric psychiatry to children in remote locations where that specialty did not exist. I believe our success in this area is part of what made the Board like us well enough to leave us alone.

The benefits of having telemedicine in the prisons were many. One disadvantage for the inmates was that they no longer got as many weekend "vacations" from the prison to the hospital. However, from the perspective of the state, they were less frequently having to pay overtime for two or more guards required to drive a state-owned vehicle and stay at the hospital with the inmate for the whole week-end or duration of their stay! Money was saved, there were fewer risks, and fewer physicians were being injured or attacked by inmates. The inmates were still receiving the care they deserved within the required 24-hour period.

We developed and filed for a patent on our Texas Department of Criminal Justice telemedicine system, but Oscar Boultinghouse made the decision that we should never enforce that patent. His thinking was that it would be better for the field of telemedicine if those patents, methods, and ideas were generally available to any practice. The papers we wrote, and the methods we developed, would play a role in both the growth of telemedicine, and in the long slow process of educating the bureaucrats and boards of the efficacy and value for this innovative and efficient delivery system for care.

— G. Byron Brooks, EE, MD

CHAPTER 5

Jay H. Sanders, MD, FACP

Johnny Appleseed

Hello darkness my old friend,
I've come to talk with you again.
Because a vision softly creeping,
left its seeds while I was sleeping...
— Paul Simon

Several times throughout this book, we refer to Jay Sanders as carrying the torch and planting the seeds of telemedicine. It was a slow process, and from the previous chapters, the reader can see that historic events were swirling around the growth of this idea. Sanders, like Johnny Appleseed, planted the seeds that would ultimately sprout and become an industry, as well as an accepted way of practicing medicine.

Throughout his career, Doctor Sanders worked to build programs, wrote papers, gave lectures and visited medical schools. By the early 90s, some of those seeds were beginning to sprout.

The Formation of the American Telemedicine Association (ATA)

In April of 1993, a group of eight physicians and one Physician Assistant formed the nonprofit incorporation, the American Telemedicine Association, or ATA. These eight doctors were Ace Allen, James Logan, Jack Moncrief, Jane Preston, Eric Tangalos, Daniel Ward, Jay Wheeler, and me, and Jim Reid the PA. None of us had known each other previously, but each was aware of each other's interest and/or involvement with telemedicine. We elected Jane Preston to serve as our first president for a two-year term.

About four to six months after the founding of the ATA, Jane brought Jonathan Linkous, a consultant from Issue Dynamics Incorporated (IDI), who made it his project to develop the ATA into an official organization. Initially, he convinced his clients at IDI to pay for his hours at the ATA, along with some help from CEO Sam Simon. In 1995, when I became the second President of the ATA, I felt that we were stable enough as an organization to hire Jonathan Linkous away from IDI and make him the first CEO of the ATA. Our first conference in 1995, was hosted by Eric Tangalos at the Mayo Clinic in Rochester, Minnesota as well as in Jacksonville, FL Bernard Harris, a graduate of Mayo Clinic and who was an astronaut on the International Space Station, did a telemedicine consultation down to us while we were having our first conference! This was how Bernard Harris got interested in telemedicine and eventually came to start Vesalius Ventures, Inc. a venture capital firm with the goal of supporting and investing in telemedicine companies.

The Ear of the DOD

In 1995, the Assistant Secretary of Defense, Dr. Stephen Joseph, came to see our 59-site system in Georgia. Prior to that visit, Steve had not been involved in telemedicine. He had previously served as the Health Commissioner for New York City and was a pediatrician but at the urging of the Chairman of the Armed Services Committee, Senator Sam Nunn, and probably also by one of the representatives from the state of Georgia, Newt Gingrich, he came to see our telemedicine program in Georgia, which was still the only state-wide telemedicine system in the US.

In those days, before PowerPoint, I would give a presentation to visitors on our system using old-fashioned slides in a conference room next to Fran Tedesco's office. When you're presenting, it's usually quite easy to see who is paying attention and engaged in what you have to say and who is, shall we say, not that interested. Well, it was clear to me that Steve did not seem that interested, and that he had probably come to see the system, not of his own volition, but due to the coercion or Congressmen Nunn and Gingrich. When I finished the slide presentation, I typically would give a live demonstration of the telemedicine system in action, which was set up in a room adjacent to the emergency department at the Medical College of Georgia.

As Steve and I were walking over to the ER, we discovered that we had been residents in Boston at the same time—he had been a pediatric resident at Boston Children's Hospital while I had been a medical resident at Massachusetts General Hospital. On this day, one of our rural hospital ER nurses had called in with a patient in the emergency department (ED) from a rural hospital in

Eastman, Georgia. This patient's complaints and reasons for being in the ED had nothing to do with his ears, but I thought to myself that, being a pediatrician, Dr. Joseph must have looked into a lot of children's ears. I saw this as the perfect opportunity to demonstrate the system. I knew that he had never seen anything like the technology that we had developed with the help of the bio-engineering department, to couple a camera to an otoscope, then transmit that image to our monitor.

I asked the patient if it would be alright if we looked inside his ear, and he obliged. The nurse put the otoscope into the patient's ear, and I smiled as I watched Steve's jaw drop to the floor.

"My God!" He exclaimed, "I have never seen a tympanic membrane that well before in my life!"

He then turned to Colonel Gomez, if I recall correctly, who was accompanying Dr. Joseph and said, "Do you know what we could do with this in the military?"

It was at that point that I knew we had "the *ear* of the DOD." And, as previously mentioned, we had also received interest from Lieutenant Colonel Fred Goeringer, the head of the Medical Advanced Technology Management Office (MATMO). He had become interested when we came up with the idea for "at home" telemedicine using the patient's TV. Through this visit in 1995 from Steve Joseph, the Department of Defense became heavily involved with and enthusiastic about telemedicine. MATMO was often referred to as the DOD "Telemedicine Test Bed."

In 1996, the interest of MATMO in telemedicine resulted in General Russ Zaitchuk, then the commanding General at Fort Detrick, asking me if they could fold their yearly medical conference into the ATA meeting.

The Umbilical Cord and the Three Musketeers

During the Clinton Administration in 1996, I was asked by Vice President Gore's office to attend a conference in Pretoria, South Africa, as a healthcare representative of the United States. Some of the other members of the delegation were Reed Hundt, named by President Clinton as the Head of the Federal Communications Commission (FCC), and Mort Bahr, the President of the Communications Workers of America. The goal of this conference was to determine how the developed nations could help the developing nations utilize communications technology to advance their health, education, and industrial infrastructure. The Health and Communication Ministers of the developing nations would be in attendance and broadcasting to South Africa.

At this conference, I remember discussing the concept of telemedicine with the Health Minister of South Africa. He pointed out to me that South Africa could not do telemedicine because they simply didn't have the communication infrastructure to support it. Having worked with rural parts of the United States to set up telemedicine, this was not foreign to me!

He continued, saying, "When we bury copper wire in the ground, within 24-48 hours, it's stolen!"

Apparently, copper being a very expensive and sought-after material, was being stolen from the ground and then sold on the black market. Ironically, during our conversation, the health minister was interrupted by one of his assistants to inform him he had a cell phone call.

When he returned from his call, he continued explaining to me how South Africa did not have the infrastructure to support telemedicine. I said to him politely, "Sir, I believe you do have the infrastructure! You just got a cellphone call!"

While nothing significant developed for South Africa at that time, it was also on this trip that Red Hundt, Mort Bahr and I became acquainted. When I told them what I was doing in telemedicine, they both became quite interested. Those relationships would later become important in the string of events that would propel telemedicine forward.

Interestingly, a decade later, Teladoc would bring telemedicine to South Africa, through a recognized entrepreneur and businessman Reg Magennis. Through the support of Magennis, Teladoc gained the full support of the phone company—using cellular structure exclusively.

Darkness

Sanford Greenberg, known as "Sandy," was the head of the Rural Healthcare Corporation, and was passionate about bringing quality healthcare access to rural America. As Zell Miller had impressed upon me, this was an immensely important task! Sandy's involvement in healthcare was the reason that he, too, caught wind of my work in telemedicine, and desired to get involved.

A great little side-story on Sandy Greenberg that is worth mentioning happened while he attended Columbia University in New York. In Sandy's junior year of college, he lost his eyesight due to glaucoma, which had been misdiagnosed. During that period, his roommate was none other than Art Garfunkel, one half of the beloved folk duo, that would later become Simon and Garfunkel. It was Art who urged and encouraged his friend, Sandy, to return to college and continue his course work. Art was a fierce friend to Sandy, nicknaming himself "the darkness," sometimes reading to him, and once, even abandoning his blind friend to navigate the subway by himself to return from Midtown to Columbia's campus.

The story goes that the friends had been out and about, and when it was time for them to return to the university, Art told Sandy he was sorry, but he had an appointment and could not go back to campus with him. Sandy was seemingly left alone to navigate Grand Central Station at rush hour in utter blind darkness. Unbeknownst to Sandy, Art was just a few paces away from him the whole time, watching to ensure the safety of his friend. When Sandy finally arrived back at campus, someone tapped him on the shoulder and said, "Excuse me, sir." It was the familiar voice of his friend, Art.

"See, I knew you could do it!" Art said, then confessed he had been with him all along. He simply wanted to prove to his friend that he could, in fact, navigate the busy New York City subway system, despite his blindness.

Eventually, Sandy would return Art's help by providing financial support to him and Paul Simon to get started. Some speculate that "The Sound of Silence" was inspired by Art Garfunkel's blind college roommate and dear friend, Sandy, but the song was, in fact, written by Paul Simon who has described its inspiration coming from his childhood habit of shutting himself in his dark bathroom to play music. Still, one must think that the inspiration and financial support from Art's old friend, nicknamed "darkness," had to play a role in the formation of the lyrics.

Sandy has dedicated much of his career to the search for the cure to blindness. He is an incredibly good, kind, generous, eternally optimistic human being, and I had the privilege of knowing him as a friend as we worked together on our mutual passion for delivering healthcare to rural America.

The 1996 Telecommunications Act scrapped several restrictions against telecommunications companies attempting to bring infrastructure to rural communities. After this, Reed Hundt established the Universal Service Administrative Company (USAC) in 1996, and the multi-billion-dollar Universal Service Fund in 1997, which enabled the FCC to stimulate the development of communication infrastructure in rural America and allowed telecommunications companies to be competitive in rural areas. The rural healthcare component received

$300 million of this funding. Schools, libraries, and high-cost, low-income areas got the bulk of the fund. Reed asked me to be chairman of the Rural Healthcare Committee and put me on the Board of Directors at the USAC, a role on which I gladly served for 15 years.

Reed, Mort Bahr, Sandy, and I worked together on this initiative to bring healthcare to rural America, but Reed, Mort, and Sandy were the "three musketeers" who truly made it happen. The transfusion from the umbilical cord of the Universal Service Fund was just what the country needed to make the delivery of healthcare to rural America a priority. To this day, the USAC's fund allows us to connect urban areas to rural areas and bring access to healthcare, and with it, convenience, decreased costs, and quite literally lives saved.

CHAPTER 6

Michael S. Gorton, MS, JD

The Unicorns of Kilimanjaro

We choose to go to the moon,
Not because it is easy,
But because it is hard
— John Kennedy

People often ask me why I climb mountains. Some assume it is a love of nature. I do love nature, but that is not why I climb. We run marathons and we climb mountains because they are hard. When we set a difficult goal like this, we must work, train, prepare and then endure whatever that mountain and nature decide to throw at us. Climbing mountains builds character and teaches us things we may not have guessed before we took that first upward step. Life is hard, particularly for a serial entrepreneur. Everything we can do to help us prepare for the challenges ahead is worth doing.

My recommendation: run marathons and climb mountains.

Kilimanjaro and Telemedicine

Gina Fidnick a schoolteacher, Chris Phelan a world-class athlete, Neecie Moore a psychologist physician, and G. Byron Brooks a former NASA Space Systems Engineer medical doctor and flight surgeon—this was the team of four friends I gathered to climb Kilimanjaro with me in the summer of 2000.

In January 2000, I sold Internet Global, a company I had started in 1992. The liquidity event had made enough money so I could pay for everyone's training, equipment, plane tickets, and satellite gear so we could communicate with family back home. We hired one of Kilimanjaro's most experienced guides: Julius Minja, and a team of porters to make sure we had the best chances of everyone reaching the summit. In the spring of 2000, the team went on several training expeditions, climbing mountains, running long distance, skiing and team building to prepare for what would be one of the most epic adventures of our lifetime.

In June, Dr. Brooks and I flew to Switzerland ahead of the team. We wanted to take a shot at climbing the Matterhorn in Switzerland. The trip to Zermatt, Switzerland, a town where no automobiles are allowed, and the climb was exhilarating.

The team, which we called vAdventures, met us in Zurich, and from there, we flew down to Nairobi, Kenya. Unfortunately, Chris Phelan's gear did not arrive, so we found ourselves in Moshi, Tanzania, buying used cold weather gear and provisions for Chris's summit attempt. Because of the caliber of athlete, Chris was probably the best person to not have his gear, but he was also the least experienced climber on the team, so it did impact his confidence ...in the beginning.

The first few days of the climb were strenuous hiking, learning Swahili, and singing traditional African songs. As we were climbing, it seemed to me that something clicked in my childhood best friend, Byron, the electrical engineer, MD. At the time, he was weaving in and out of his work in correctional care at the University of Texas Medical Branch in Galveston (UTMB), and flight surgeon job. I found it strange that he didn't talk about it much. Was it possible he had become bored with it?

I believe that when he realized his serial entrepreneur friend had built something that had made more money than he ever could have made in a nine-to-five job, he felt competitive and inspired. In reality, everything Byron and I did was competitive. It was a great virtue that drove many successful summits over the years. As we trekked the tallest mountain in Africa, he began making suggestions that we needed to build a company.

Always searching for and reaching toward the next goal, I asked, "Okay, Byron. Hit me. Whadda ya got?"

"Well, I am doing this telemedicine thing..." he began. He described telemedicine rooms in every city in America and across the globe, where a patient could be connected to any doctor via telemedicine and could put on a vest that would take and send their vitals to the doctor. And he wanted to call it Cyber Medical Services. Immediately, I could see that was not going to work. For one thing, it would be way too expensive to get one of these special telemedicine rooms in every city across the US, but also, *The Terminator* movies taught me we didn't want cyber *anything!* The truth is the name he wanted almost made me NOT want to build it.

Meanwhile, the porters from our expedition and others had caught on that Byron was a doctor and, nightly, there was a line of Tanzanians outside his tent, coming to him with their medical complaints, and Byron would tell them what to do. Funny side story,—they all called him "kaka." In the US, that was a childhood word for…uhh, excrement. Alas, kaka is Swahili for "brother," but the new nickname did add some fun to the expedition.

Besides treating the guides and porters, I noticed Byron using technology to communicate over the course of our expedition to treat patients back in the States.

"Byron," I asked him, "Are you taking consults from back home?"

"Yeah," he answered. It was simple, and matter of fact.

"Now that is a business model! When we get back to the States, we need to talk about *that*," I said.

After four days of hiking up on one of the world's largest mountains, we had reached the camp a mile below the summit. The final summit attempt for a mountain like Kilimanjaro typically begins by waking up around midnight. On the morning of June 15, 2000, the five of us, accompanied by our two guides, broke camp and departed Arrow Campground just after midnight with an outside temperature of about minus twenty Fahrenheit. We slowly made our way up the ice falls, then up a steep scree embankment.

It was hard.

The air was thin.

Have I mentioned that it was hard? It was really hard!

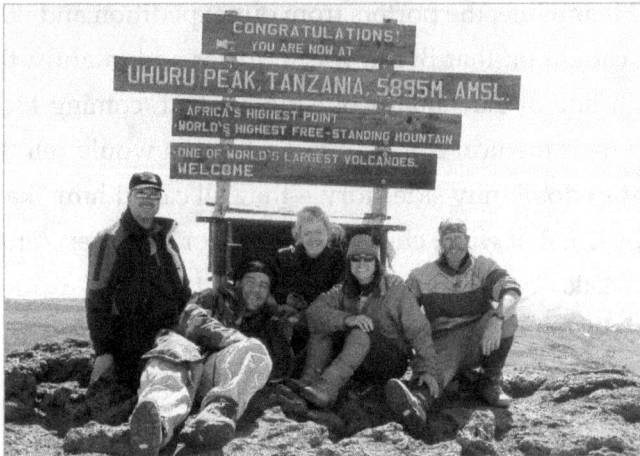

Michael Gorton, Byron Brooks, MD, Neecie Moore, Gina Fidnick, and Chris Phelan

There were times when we would count twenty steps, then rest.

The entire team reached the summit. Chris, who was climbing in secondhand gear, made it look easy. He even did a hundred push-ups on the peak that day! We all made it back down, enjoyed an amazing four days on photographic safari in Tanzania, then returned to the States.

Spoiler alert, Byron and I found a Unicorn on Kilimanjaro. It was cleverly disguising itself as a creature called Cyber Medical Services and evading us through the hard work of reaching the summit. To this day, I believe there are more Unicorns on that mountain. Someday, I will return to Kilimanjaro with my kids. Perhaps we will find another Unicorn, but either way, the adventure with the kids will be worth the effort.

Unicorn is an entrepreneur term for a company that reaches a net-worth of more than a billion dollars. In the early 2000s, Unicorns were almost nonexistent. Today, they are still incredibly rare. The company I had sold prior to Kilimanjaro was valued at $122 million, and that was almost front-page news.

I hadn't gone to Kilimanjaro thinking about building a new company, and if I was going to build another company, it was going to be with Dr. Neecie Moore, the entrepreneurial psychologist physician, on our trip. Neecie and I had connected in the north Texas entrepreneurial network and the two of us were consulting and building a fairly large number of companies. Internet Global, the company I had just sold, was an internet and telecommunications company—about as far from healthcare as it could be, or so I thought.

Long before Byron and I decided to climb Kili, Jay Sanders had planted the telemedicine seed with Oscar Boultinghouse, a physician at UTMB. The potential around that opportunity had grown in the mind of Byron, the electrical engineer, MD, who thought he wanted to be an entrepreneur.

It is always interesting how things come together. I was pondering all these elements when I came back to the States after nearly a month in Europe and Africa. I decided to get together with Nathan Morton, a great personal mentor who knew how to take an idea and build it into a billion-dollar Unicorn.

Nathan's personal story was a great one that played an

important role in the formation and growth of Teladoc. In his early career, he had been the manager of a small department store with just a few locations. He looked around and saw how well it was being run and thought, *this store could be everywhere.*

Morton contacted the owners of that store, called Target and said, "I have this idea. I know how to take this store and turn it into 200 stores in just a couple of years."

The owners liked his idea and said, "Let's do it!"

Obviously, his plan was successful. *Business Week* wrote an article about him, and with that, another store owner from Atlanta called him and said, "I want to do the same thing with my hardware store!"

Long story short, it was Nathan's vision that helped Home Depot become what it is today. After that, he received a call from a nerd who had a small computer store in Dallas called Software House. Nathan Morton told him, "I want to build it as the CEO and call it CompUSA."

And so he did. Right after growing CompUSA past the $4 billion mark, I managed to spark his interest and get a meeting with him. It is a pretty scary day when a young sergeant's kid gets to meet with a great titan of business, like Nathan Morton.

Nathan and I became friends, and he agreed to help me build Internet Global, the company I ultimately sold, which paid my way to Kilimanjaro.

Upon my return to the States from Africa, I was having

lunch with Nathan, and I told him, "I am thinking about building a telemedicine company."

After I described it to him, he told me, "You need to do this!"

You definitely need to do this!

Having Nathan affirm this idea was extraordinary, because everyone else I had talked to about it had told me it was a stupid idea. Nathan was insistent. "It's not a Dallas company. It's not a Texas company. Turn it into something the whole country and ultimately the world knows about. If you do this right, you will build something that will be worth more than what I built at CompUSA."

"Okay, but *how* do I do it?" I asked him. The thought of building a company worth more than $4 billion seemed insanely impossible, but this was Nathan Morton advising me, so I believed it.

Thus, the real mentoring began. Essentially, what he told me is that you must begin with the end in mind. If you want to live in a mansion, but you only lay the foundation for a tiny cottage, you'll end up having to tear the walls down, re-pour the foundation, and start over each time you grow. Nathan told me envision the company as it would be in five years and pour the foundation for the mansion. Once I knew what I was building, I could figure out how to get the resources, and more importantly, he advised me to get the best assets we possibly could.

From the beginning, the idea was met with resistance.

First, I called Jay Sanders and asked him to be an advisor. We had no traction, and our emphasis was more on telephone-medical consults, rather than video and technical data collection. Doctor Sanders said "no." It wasn't until four years later, when we started making waves, that he finally took my call and agreed.

I needed money to build this company, so the next thing I did was begin to call the investors for whom I had just made a lot of money. Left and right, they were telling me, "No," "Stupid idea," and, "Not interested."

I called an investor who made about 50 times his money on an investment in my former company, Internet Global, and he told me no. Another one, named Gary, was telling me no, and I reminded him he had written a check to Internet Global and made a significant return. With some coercion, Gary agreed to write us a check for $25,000. Seventeen years later, in the spring of 2021, I called him to ask if he had sold his stock yet. He told me that, yes, he had just sold it, and that he had made north of $5 million!

Since almost all the investors I called told me no, I knew I was going to have to get scrappy. The next thing I did was to call all the people who had worked for me at Internet Global who had made money on their stock. One of the first people I called was my programmer, Derek, from Internet Global.

"I'd love to help you, Michael," he said, "But I've got a great job. I am not willing to give it up for a startup. Why don't you talk to Michelle, my wife, who is an even better programmer than I am."

At first, I was skeptical. Michelle was four foot something tall and seemed quiet. I could not picture her running IT for me. It didn't take long before I realized just how good Michelle was. She was a force of nature, and one of the many essential puzzle pieces that made Teladoc a success. A few years after we hired her, her husband Derek also came to work for us. He had to take a job reporting to his wife! Gotta love that one.

There would be several other key team members who I would call to join us. I would remind them how successful we had been at Internet Global and tell them we couldn't pay them well. Still, they chose to add their talents to the mix. I think something like 20 or 30 people bet on the potential and began working at this telemedicine startup making almost nothing. It was truly inspirational to see people adopting and joining the dream.

The bottom line is a reiteration of the adage that necessity is the mother of invention. We started Teladoc with a great idea, less than a million dollars, and a lot of sweat equity. As we were beginning to grow the model, Chuck May introduced me to Bruce Quinnell. Bruce is one of the clearest thinkers I had ever met. He made an investment and joined the Board alongside Nathan Morton. Over the years, I would come to see Quinnell as one of the best resources and friends of my lifetime. He gets a lot of credit for helping us plow through some of the nearly impossible tasks.

Now we had a team, a great board, and an idea, but what was next? What did we need? There was no national network of doctors, no electronic medical record, there was no call center that could do this, no billing system capable of this task. We didn't have an interface or any knowledge of how to deal with the Blue Crosses, Uniteds, Cignas, or Aetnas (then called BUCAs) of the world. What does the business model look like? Who joins? How do they join? What do they pay?

This was a mountain far taller and more difficult than Kilimanjaro, where the idea was born.

A Note on Successful Entrepreneurism

The task list sounds almost insurmountable, but solving problems like this is the nature of being an entrepreneur. I have had plenty of friends in corporate America who had an idea and come to me for advice. Should they quit their job and build a company? Mostly I tell them not to do it. Changing the world is not about great ideas. It is about implementation, hard work, and (often) getting knocked down and kicked in the teeth. There are great people in corporate America, but the skills are different for the entrepreneur.

Success as an entrepreneur starts with an idea. It is funny to me how many people have told me one or many of the companies I have built was really their idea. They thought of it long before I had started building it. Saying I want to climb a mountain does not get me to the summit. We have to begin with the idea. Without the initial idea, there is nothing.

Ideas are easy compared to the grind of turning them into reality.

The next important element is building the plan. This goes back to what Nathan Morton was telling us earlier in this chapter. If you want to change the world, think BIG. As my friend Allen West is always saying, if you set the bar low, you will never jump high.

After the plan, and the big dream is in place, you have to find the people who can help build it. My personal philosophy is in alignment with the great Stephen Covey: Trust and Inspire. Surround yourself with smart people, give them a piece of the company, trust them, and inspire them. When you make the dream into their dream, there is nothing they won't do to make sure it comes to fruition.

If you are the leader in a company, you need to leave your ego at home. Companies and great ideas fail when egos enter the work environment. This is an important point, so I will say it another way. Ego is a lethal poison. Make sure it does not come into your Teladoc. Over the years, Bruce Quinnell and I became good friends. We often debated issues in the boardroom. Generally, he was right, and as a result, I learned. The important thing is that we left our egos at the door. We had a fiduciary responsibility to make the right decisions for our company, not the ones that made us feel powerful.

The final fundamental element of a successful startup is persistence. I love the Calvin Coolidge quote on persistence and recommend it to anyone thinking about building a world changing company.

Nothing in the world can take the place of persistence. Talent will not; nothing is more common than unsuccessful men with talent. Genius will not; unrewarded genius is almost a proverb. Education will not; the world is full of educated derelicts. Persistence and determination alone are omnipotent.

— Calvin Coolidge

You are going to be challenged every day, and survival of your great ideal will take a lot of persistence. My favorite personal story is the first day as a freshman engineering student. The dean is addressing the entire class in a giant auditorium: "Look left and look right. Only one of you will still be here at graduation." To my left was a valedictorian and to my right, a salutatorian. I graduated #32 in my class. I wanted to be an engineer more than anything I had ever wanted, so I was terrified! I got knocked down and kicked in the teeth a lot during engineering school, but I learned that you just need to get up, put on a smile, fix the problem, and go again.

To quote Muhammad Ali: *"You don't lose if you get knocked down; you lose if you stay down."*

Some people think it takes luck. Sometimes circumstance is insurmountable, but my current company, Recuro Health, has a chairman named William Paiva, who is always telling us that luck is something we create. I tend to agree. Most of the time, people can make their own luck by being prepared, and keeping their eyes open for opportunity.

Make sure you expose yourself to every diverse position possible. You never know who you are going to meet. Interestingly, sometimes opportunity comes in the middle of the greatest difficulty. History is full of stories about people who rose above adversity, changed the world, and maybe even became famous in the process.

Keep your eyes open and don't give up. In the final chapters of this book, we will tell you about nearly impossible adversity, and how we overcame it.

If you have a great idea, you will get knocked down and kicked in the teeth – a lot. Get up, put a smile on, figure out what you did wrong and go again!

CHAPTER 7

Michael S. Gorton, MS, JD

Turning the Torch Into a Rocket Engine

They taught us in engineering school that the finest steel
is forged in fire and annealed by cooling.
— Michael Gorton

I have great admiration for my co-author Jay Sanders. He is a brilliant and fun-loving man with a kind heart. When I recently asked him to work with me on this book, he said something to the effect of: "Sure, but we must hurry because I am not getting any younger!" From my point of view, Jay has maintained his health better than most. My advice is that he should not be concerned about buying green bananas.

I must admit, it upsets me when Jay says he is not the "Father of Telemedicine." I will stipulate to the fact that Dr. Ken Bird created the idea. After he cleared his initial skepticism, Jay Sanders was always front and center in the growth and nurturing of that idea. He is the man who carried the torch and planted the seeds. He is still doing exactly that.

The fire (torch) analogy is a perfect one because controlling fire is likely one of the first great innovations for humanity. Taking that fire and turning it into the force behind a rocket engine brought us to the Moon. Dr. Sanders shouted into the wind for a very long time before the innovation planted the seed that grew to the next level.

Building the Rocket Engine

On day one, we, the cofounders at Teladoc knew we had a great idea. We assembled the team and began the nearly impossible task of building the company. There was not a simple Electronic Medical Record, no national network of telemedicine doctors, no call center, no billing system, no complete book of the hodgepodge of laws in the fifty states. We had a lot to do! The fact is, we had no idea of just how much we had to do.

In conclusion, tackling impossible tasks is pretty much the case for all entrepreneurs when they begin the journey of building a company that is destined to change the world.

At the time, most primary care physicians (PCPs) were exhausted from working long hours with low income. Our internal poll showed PCPs were working in excess of sixty hours per week and making about $148,000. Certainly, that is a decent pay, but with the workload, responsibility over life itself, caliber of people who make it into and through medical school, then work sixty hours per week—it should be a lot more. With the constant rising costs of care, it seems crazy to advocate for anyone to make more, but that is exactly what I was thinking. Doctors should make more … and patients should pay less!

Many of the smartest people in undergrad went off to med school and ended in a role where they didn't have time to use their number one asset: their creative and analytical brains. Because of this, many PCPs were looking for something different. Around that time, we were seeing the beginnings of something called Concierge Medicine.

The basic model for Concierge Medicine was that a patient would pay a doctor an annual sum of money to be their "concierge doctor." The doctor and patient would meet once a year to golf, grab lunch, and assess the patient's overall health. Then, the patient had access to the doctor for any healthcare related need they had throughout the year—day or night. Suddenly, doctors who were working insane hours, making $140,000, and treating patients nonstop all day were able to spend time with their patients, and could make around $250,000-450,000 a year depending on the number of concierge patients!

Pricing Model

Dr. Brooks and I studied the Concierge Medicine model when we were thinking about building the business model for Teladoc. We thought about charging patients $100 a month to do a telemedicine version of the Concierge model. Patients could use the system as much as they wanted without additional charges. We did not have much success and continued playing with different models until we came up with $1 dollar a month and $35 per consult. The average PCP visit was $110, so this model made sense. As it turned out, this was the pricing model that worked and launched the telemedicine industry.

An important element in the pricing was understanding the concept of utilization. If a company is paying per employee per month (PEPM), how much are the employees using the service? In the beginning, employee subscribers did not know what telemedicine was, and utilization was pretty low. Understanding conditions that supported very low utilization gave us the ability to give special pricing to resellers, brokers, and some companies.

In the early years of Teladoc, a seasoned, healthcare trained sales and marketing executive named Gary Wald decided to join us. Gary and I were trying to find that first big customer. We were focused on a national reseller called New Benefits, run by Joel Ray. After several meetings, we knew we were getting close. On the day we thought we would get Joel to say yes, his administrative assistant called to cancel because he was sick.

At first, I was distraught. But then, the entrepreneur kicked in!

Working with the premise of polite persistence, I was determined to see Joel. I knew because of his work ethic and dedication, he would be in the office (sick or not), so Gary and I barged in—politely. His administrative assistant tried to stop us, but persistence won out on that day, as we coerced our way into the CEO's office. We told Joel this was the perfect test for the Teladoc model!

"I have a friend who is a doctor. I have already called him and am awaiting his return call," Joel informed us.

"Perfect," I said. "Your friend has not called back, so let's sign you up for Teladoc and run a comparison."

Joel agreed, and the Teladoc physician called in under

an hour. His doctor friend called the next morning. Same diagnosis, same prescription. Joel was in!

Joel Ray's New Benefits company was our first large account, but they were also the experts on pricing and utilization. From Joel, we learned much about how to price in a win-win scenario. Much of what we learned from those lessons is still in effect throughout telemedicine today.

SuperDoc and the 3-Hour Guarantee

Something valuable that Dr. Brooks contributed was his understanding, in advance, of the problems we would have to address. Corporate practice of medicine was a minefield. The doctors could not work for me or Teladoc Inc., the company, because I am not a doctor. The practice of medicine correctly, does not want capitalism, CEOs and non-physicians dictating diagnosis and treatment. That job should be done by trained medical doctors outside of the influence of capitalism.

Our solution was to create an independent Physicians Association called Teladoc, PA. Teladoc, Inc. handled accounting, electronic medical records, and patient acquisition, along with all the other technology and connectivity elements. The physicians joined the PA with the primary job of handling the consult. I ran the corporate (membership) entity, while Bruce Begia, MD and Roger Moczygemba, MD ran the PA.

The goal was always to make it very simple for the physician and the patient.

As mentioned before, PCPs were working crazy hours and only taking home an average of $148K. We soon realized that we could give those PCPs the opportunity to work forty hours per week, any time of day they wanted, and increase their income by $100,000. That's right—a doctor could work forty hours from home and make $250,000. More importantly, they could spend more time with the patient, listen, analyze, and diagnose. There is a lesson every doctor learns in med school: "Listen to your patients and they will tell you what is wrong." The Teladoc engine gave the providers more time to spend with the patient so they could listen. They made more money in the process, and had more free time to learn, spend time with their family and enjoy life. As we said back then, we changed the efficiency paradigm in care delivery.

As we were developing the patient populations to support full-time work for the doctors, we had to find physicians willing to try the telemedicine delivery method. Dr. Begia had a few doctors at the Alamo City Medical group who could cover us when we were testing in the state of Texas, but as we expanded nationwide, recruiting became critical. Shelley Laine and Lisa Fletcher began attending physician conferences to recruit and teach about the benefits of telemedicine. Our business model required all physicians to be board certified, which narrowed the number of prospects. Even though our delivery system was new, our PA worked to define the highest standards.

Looking back, I recall an amazing amalgamation of

doctors in the PA. Many physicians who were retiring from the daily grind, but still wanted to practice on their own time, joined us. We had a few doctors who had been in accidents and were no longer ambulatory. One of my favorites came from a married couple. She was an anesthesiologist, and he was a PCP. When their baby was born, he stayed home and joined Teladoc PA. The family income went up!

In the beginning, Teladoc gave members a guarantee that we would deliver a doctor in three hours, or Teladoc Inc. would pay for the $35 consult. Note that the telemedicine doc was paid because we assumed our engine would make the connection in that three-hour window. It was a scary proposition, but we almost never had to fulfill that "free consult" guarantee. By 2006, we were delivering doctors to patients in about twelve minutes, nationwide!

There were states around the country where we had just a few members. It is difficult to inspire a physician to join the PA when they only have the opportunity to do a couple of consults per year. We solved that problem by creating something we called the SuperDoc program. With SuperDoc, we offered to do all the work and pay all the licensing fees for our providers who wanted to be multistate licensed. It was a huge success, increasing physician revenue, decreasing response time, and improving access in low-volume states.

So, how was it that doctors were working fewer hours and making more money? Think about the primary care office that you visit when you are sick. The expense list starts with a building, waiting room, admin, phone system, computers, equipment, doctors, nurses, etc... That is a powerful engine and definitely overkill for treating minor issues.

A favorite analogy is like discovering fire ants in your front yard, calling the Pentagon and asking them to send a brigade, tanks and fighter aircraft! Calling in the US Army to treat fire ants seemed to fit the analogy of treating minor issues with a fully equipped medical practice.

It is a simple equation—treat only minor issues. Cut virtually all of your costs. Charge the patient less money. The end result, believe it or not, is the doctor makes more!

Simplicity is everything. In science, we have a principle called Occam's Razor, which teaches the scientist that the simplest solution is generally the correct one. An application of Occam's Razor is something we seldom do in healthcare.

Navigating the Quagmire of Regulations

From the very beginning, Dr. Brooks was educating and cautioning about the potential land mines associated with the regulatory environment. I mentioned the Corporate Practice of Medicine above, but there was a lot more. Each state had its own set of laws, so a practice operating in all fifty states needed to know the rules, times fifty!

We made a decision on day one to NOT allow the system to treat issues that required controlled substances. We built our engine around that principle. It became a part of our training tools for our members and our doctors. Our goal was to design a fool-proof system where it simply could not happen. Our solution was elegant and simple. The doctor's role was to treat the patient and update the medical record. If a prescription was issued, the burden of calling in the script was removed from the doctor. We hired a team of nurses to call in the prescriptions. That lightened the doctor's workload, but it also gave the nurse team the ability to make sure the PA and Teladoc Inc. had that second layer of protection. I believe it is safe to say that we never prescribed a narcotic or other Drug Enforcement Agency (DEA) regulated substance.

In most states, doctors had tight restrictions on their ability to advertise. That included web pages, so most practices just avoided it all together. For Teladoc, we worked diligently to make sure our website did not cross the line. Because our website could be seen in all fifty states, our objective was to design it to comply with the strictest state regulations.

Fee splitting is another regulation that we studied closely. As we built our business model, we recognized that the doctors working for us could not split that $35 consult fee with Teladoc, Inc. We navigated this problem by having Inc. provide accounting for the PA. All consult fees were collected at the PA, and Inc. billed the PA for the various services like accounting, call center, and maintenance of electronic medical records. Our profits in the Inc. came from the per member per month (PMPM) fee. Note that in a company environment, this is often done per employee, so you have a PEPM in that scenario. A simple way of saying this is that Teladoc Inc. was a membership organization. Our members had the benefit of exclusive access to the Teladoc Physicians Association.

In the beginning, we hoped that there would be some degree of reciprocity of licenses across state lines. What I mean by this comes down to a simple question: is it appropriate for a New York licensed doctor to treat a Colorado patient? In our current system, this is not a biological question, but a regulatory one. Of course, the reader is welcome to crack any jokes about the residents of their neighboring states. Because Bill Giles, my CFO, was from Oklahoma, he and I often did!

In the beginning, we wanted to understand reciprocity and interstate medicine in great detail. Later, we abandoned it altogether. More on this issue in the next chapter, but we just could not find a pathway. Even with bordering states, we decided to never practice across state lines.

Practicing across state lines becomes more complex when you realize that a Texas resident who is visiting Florida must be treated by a doctor licensed in Florida. When a patient came into the queue, we knew their home state because of their membership, but we always asked where they currently were. We refined this model so well that we could treat interstate truckers. For them, we would find out which highway and direction, then do the calculus for where they would be when the prescription was called in.

We even researched to find a pharmacy that had a parking lot capable of accommodating an 18-wheeler!

In the beginning, no states addressed telemedicine in their Legislative Code. It was our huge task to find out a much more fundamental question. How did the Code address a physician treating a patient she had never touched? This became the fundamental issue blocking the practice of telemedicine. We needed to develop a solution to regulatory resistance on this question. Could it ever be appropriate for a physician to treat a patient they have never touched?

Finding answers to all the regulatory questions was a seemingly insurmountable burden for a startup company that had raised less than a couple of million dollars. We asked our law firm to see if there was an existing document that addressed the legal questions for all fifty states. The law firm happily informed us that no such document existed. They proposed creating one, a task that would take six months and cost us something like a quarter million dollars.

WOW! That is not good news for a startup company.

I called Grant Seabolt, an investor and one of my former law school professors, to see if he had any creative suggestions. From that call came not only a Teladoc caliber efficiency solution, but a lifelong friendship.

Rocky Dhir was a licensed attorney, building a practice called Atlas Legal. Rocky hired US and UK educated lawyers living in India to use Lexus and Westlaw for research. Because the cost of living and wages were so much lower in India, the model worked. Rocky's team produced the first 50-state definitive manual answering all the legal questions I have addressed. Rocky and his state-side legal team of licensed attorneys reviewed the research and produced the book. The best news is that the Atlas Legal team finished the project in a couple of weeks for about $16,000!

Mechanics of the Teladoc Model

So, how does an engine that delivers doctors to patients in fifty states in well under three hours work? When we started the company, all doctors had pagers. No one had smart phones. Video conferencing technology existed, but only engineers and geeks knew how to use it. We did test video, along with email—now known as asynchronous consults. No one used them.

The engine worked like this:
1. Patient dials into the call center.
2. Call center makes sure the caller is a member, where they currently are, and their preferred pharmacy.
3. Call center moves patient to a queue that notifies all physicians who are signed in and licensed to practice in the state from which the patient is calling.
4. The first doctor to pull the patient from the queue wins. I say "wins" because it becomes a race. This

is the bullet that got us to a 12-minute response time! It literally became a race.

5. Physician reviews patient's medical history, and chief complaint, then calls the patient.
6. After the consult is complete, the doctor updates and closes the medical record.
7. If the consult generated a prescription, the on-call nurses are notified to review, and call in the script.
8. Every patient is asked to do a quick survey after the consult.

The patient satisfaction surveys mentioned in #8 above were created and administered by one of the great thought leaders in healthcare, Arnie Milstein at Mercer. We were consistently seeing over 95% satisfaction with the service. No other entity delivering care was coming anywhere close to those numbers. It was, in fact, that level of satisfaction that inspired former HHS Secretary Tommy Thompson to join our Advisory group. Like many others, Governor Thompson became an essential asset to the company, and a lifelong friend to me.

After several years of developing applications, testing and tweaking, it was time to grow. Gary Wald conducted a nationwide search for a PR firm that could handle our needs. Laura Carabello, founder of the New Jersey firm CPR, won the bid. I can only describe Laura's results one way: startlingly great. We did our press release in May 2005. Over the course of the next seven months, the CPR team produced over seven hundred mainstream PR events. I appeared on almost every television talk show. Major publications like the *New York Times, Wall Street Journal,* and almost every major city newspaper ran stories. For clarity, this new thing called Teladoc was controversial. Many of the articles were negative, suggesting we should be shut down. A scary number demanded that management should be imprisoned! Some predicted an avalanche of bad outcomes and malpractice would result from telemedicine. We quickly learned how new ideas are met with resistance. Still, I believe the majority of the articles were cautiously positive.

Sometime around January 2006, I had to call Laura and the CPR team to request they stop. I had been spending too much time communicating with the press while our telemedicine company was experiencing exponential growth.

As the member population was approaching two million in 2008 and 2009, I decided that John Halsey's architectural advice on how to grow the company had worked. John was the one who knew healthcare and designed our pathway from small company customers through the ecosystem of brokers, TPAs, enterprise self-insureds, up to the elusive payers. To be fair, it took a significant number of smart experts to get us to that two million number. I think about people like Bruce Quinnell, Carl Dickerson, Tommy Thompson, Bob Kramer, Richard Lungen, Jeff Gary, and so many others who all worked as a team to get us that first major BUCA contract.

Sadly, during the growth period, we lost the great Nathan Morton, who advised me to proceed when all others called it stupid. Nathan was a founding Board member along with Bruce Quinnell and was greatly missed when he died suddenly of a virus he picked up during an international trip.

CHAPTER 8

Michael S. Gorton, MS, JD

Judge, Jury, and Executioner

Whether you think you can, or
think you can't—you're right.
— Henry Ford

I have built fourteen companies. Some have had a modicum of success, and some have failed. A few have been absolute home runs, and Teladoc was more like a World Series, game winning grand slam. Even the failures bring invaluable knowledge and experience that helps the next endeavor.

In all the companies where I have raised capital, I have heard professional investors ask the question, "What keeps you up at night?"

I have always hated that one, because almost nothing ever does. Early on, I felt I had to answer the question with something that might keep me up, but then just started saying NOTHING. That was an accurate response until Teladoc.

In some ways, this is the most startling and interesting part of this story. In this chapter, you will learn why telemedicine took so long to become mainstream, and what can keep an intrepid entrepreneur up at night.

A few stories from the early days of Telemedicine

Something I learned early on is that the Boards of

Medical Examiners have their own court system, their own judges. The physicians in any given state are licensed and work at the whim of the Board of Medical Examiners. If a physician does something wrong and is called in for a hearing, sometimes the Board will take their license, sometimes they won't. Either way, it's a terrifying experience for the physician because even if they have what they believe is good evidence to support their case and an excellent lawyer, the Board has all the power. I think generally, the Boards provide an important service for the state residents, but if they are opposed to something, overcoming that opposition is borderline impossible.

Our first meeting with the Board of Medical Examiners happened in Texas about two years into Teladoc. Some of our doctors were concerned that Teladoc may not be in full compliance with the law. I naively believed the Board of Medical Examiners would support our position on this issue, so I was rather insistent with Doctor Boultinghouse and Doctor Brooks that they help me schedule a meeting with the Board, because I knew the Board would take their call. It just seemed so clear to me that we were impacting access for the patients while simultaneously improving the physician experience, revenue, and business model for the doctor.

I remember Oscar saying, "Man, you don't schedule a meeting with the Board of Medical Examiners—they schedule a meeting with *you*. And when they do, it's almost never a good thing!"

Nonetheless, we did schedule the meeting, and I went into that building in Austin, TX excited because I felt like we had something that was going to change everything! We had a couple hundred patients in Texas, and both doctor and patient alike were loving it. The doctors were getting paid well and were working fewer hours, the patients were getting rapid care, and it was saving money. Satisfaction levels on both the patient and physician side were in the stratosphere.

At our meeting, I enthusiastically told the Board all the ways Teladoc was solving problems and just how well it was working.

"Mr. Gorton," they said, "if you build this company, you will go to prison, and Doctor Brooks, we will take your license and then you'll go to prison."

I was shocked! I had been so optimistic going into this meeting, believing they would support us and cheer us on. Instead, they told us, "They would never allow doctors in the State of Texas to treat a patient they haven't touched."

We walked out of that room deflated. Oscar, who had been practicing telemedicine for some time, but always under the umbrella of a state government, immediately said, "I'm out." Byron said he thought he might be out, too. They did not want to lose their licenses over this. I spent the next few weeks trying to convince Byron not to jump ship.

At the time, Byron had served as a consultant to the Board on the topic of telemedicine. After our meeting, he returned to UTMB and received a call from the Board. They said there was this new telemedicine company in Texas called Teladoc and they wanted to know what he thought about them.

Byron was perplexed. "Wait a minute," he said. "That was me. I was there. How many black doctors practicing telemedicine do you think there are in this state?"

Here he was, helping start this company, and the Board was calling him, their consultant, asking him what he thought of the company he was helping start. He was just shocked that they hadn't made the connection that the Teladoc doctor was him.

In a debriefing with Dr. Brooks and another physician colleague, Dr. Begia, we made a fundamental realization that would ultimately pave the way for those Boards willing to be reasonable. Doctors commonly used something called cross coverage. Doctor Jones cannot work 24-hours per day, so he works with his colleague Doctor Smith to "cover" on Tuesday and Thursday. In this scenario, Doctor Smith will receive calls from Jones's patient, who she has never met.

The Board was fine with the cross-coverage scenario. As we saw it, cross-coverage is fundamentally broken. Dr. Smith has no way of verifying the caller is really Doctor Jones' patient. She does not get paid for the consultation. She does not have a medical record for history, and a file after the consultation.

The covering physician, who has never before touched

this patient, must make decisions on the patient's care, while the primary physician is not available. Most importantly, the Board was fine with that.

Unfortunately, I was not able to find anything in writing about cross-coverage in the literature of the Texas Board of Medical Examiners or the Texas Code. Yet, all the physicians and the Board know it's there and use it. Against all odds, Byron and I put together a case and returned to the Board of Medical examiners about six weeks after our initial meeting. In great detail, we explained to them how what we were doing at Teladoc was cross-coverage, and that we were even improving it!

We explained that cross coverage was really just a collegial, shaking of hands, saying, "Sure, I'll cover for you!" There were many flaws in this system. There was no pay associated with it for the covering physician, and the covering physician rarely had access to the patient's medical records. If the covering physician treated a patient, there was no way it was making it into the medical record. And if they made a mistake, they could be sued. Usually, what cross-coverage meant for the patient is that, if they had a minor issue like a cold, it would have to wait until the primary physician was back on Monday. If there was a more serious problem, the covering physician would then jump through hoops to ensure the patient was cared for. So, from the patient's perspective, sometime cross-coverage worked, sometimes it didn't. From the physician's perspective, they were just doing this to help out a fellow physician—there was no real benefit to them, and often there were serious risks.

When we brought all these flaws from the acceptable standard of care (cross coverage) to the attention of the Texas Board of Medical Examiners and explained to them how Teladoc was, in fact, solving many of these problems, they gave us the go-ahead! To be sure, it was not a strong endorsement, but for my entrepreneurial mindset, it was enough.

With a soft approval from the State of Texas, we boldly chose to move forward. Over the years, I had been told that if telemedicine was viable, one of the big healthcare companies would have done it. In addition, in the years since, many people have said they had the idea long before me and therefore they should get credit for the innovation. At Teladoc, we did not create the idea. We just built the first big telemedicine platform. But I agree, any of the giants could have done it.

But they didn't. Can you imagine what one of the major payors (BUCAs) would have done if the Board had told them they could go to prison? As they say on the streets, "Enough said."

In the following stories, I think you will see why it took a team of entrepreneurs—intrepid entrepreneurs.

We faced legal challenges from seventeen states, and several other governmental entities, politicians, some of the large healthcare companies, and the press. Because telemedicine is now mainstream and accepted nationwide,

Dr. Sanders and I decided we would rather not name those states involved in the stories from this book. As the line from the old Dragnet TV show goes, the names have been changed to protect the innocent.

Hmmm, maybe innocent is not the right word. We will let you decide that one. :-)

Shortly after Texas, we started rolling service out across the United States...and, at the same time, began getting certified mail and summons from states demanding response to their "concerns" about our practice.

By the time I left Teladoc, seventeen different states challenged the practice. We always used the same strategy: we would inform them how the Texas Board had looked into Teladoc and had approved the way we were improving cross-coverage. We knew that if we showed up at the Board in any state with Lawyers, Guns, and Money, so to speak, we would lose. Instead, we developed our thought leadership, built relationships with well-known healthcare experts, and passively tried to show the Boards how telemedicine would improve care in their state.

Incidentally, my use of the phrase "Lawyers, Guns, and Money" is one I used a lot during the challenges described in this chapter. The phrase for me originated in a Warren Zevon song called: *Send Lawyers, Guns, and Money*. In the song, Zevon is asking his dad to send those things to get him out of trouble. While I loved the phrase, I was convinced that tactic would fail, so we NEVER used lawyers and money.

State A

For some states, "thought leadership" and simple explanation were good enough. Others, like State A, took a little more convincing.

State A told us we could not call what we were doing at Teladoc cross-coverage and get away with it. This led to us visiting their offices. What I remember them saying was that only a physician can define who covers for them when they are unavailable. I found that quite remarkable! We tried to take a Constitutional argument with them.

Doesn't a patient have the right to choose their doctor? Yes.

Yet, when their doctor is not available, we were being told that only the doctor can say who covers for them?

Correct.

Shouldn't the patient get a say in who covers when their primary care doctor is not available?

NO. Cross coverage is for the doctor to decide, not the patient.

The Teladoc PA believed that everyone should have a primary care doctor, and Teladoc could not fill that role. In our contract with members, every member (patient) was required to tell us who their PCP was, and to designate Teladoc as their cross-coverage doctor.

The theory behind cross coverage was simple. A patient has the right to select the primary care doctor. Teladoc was not designed to replace the PCP, only to provide convenience when that PCP was not readily available, and only to treat minor issues.

We recognized that, once a patient used the service and experienced a doctor call in minutes, that patient might want to replace their PCP with Teladoc. We built logic into the engine to inform our doctors how often the patient was calling in. There were plenty of circumstances where our doctor told the patient they must visit the PCP. By the way, we did fire a few patients for constantly trying to use Teladoc as their PCP!

We explained all these things to State A, but they held their ground. Teladoc was not cross coverage because only the PCP can designate who can serve as cross. Bad news for patients in State A! You get to select your PCP, but not who covers when that PCP is not immediately available. I recall thinking what an egregious breach of Constitutional rights!

This might have been a viable battle—using Lawyers, Guns, and Money, but I was not interested in legal battles. We had a company to build, and I knew State A would eventually come around. We stopped service in State A. They eventually came around.

State B

It was two days before Christmas and Alice Carol (name changed), a Teladoc physician and Navy reserve lieutenant, took a call. Alice was (still is, I presume) an extraordinary individual who donated about 50% of her time to providing care to indigents in State B, and the other 50% she worked in the Navy Reserves.

On the Teladoc line that night, the patient was in tears, explaining to Dr. Carol that he was in immense pain. He had run out of his oxycontin and, since it was a holiday, his doctor was on vacation until the New Year. The patient would not be able to get a refill of the drug for some time.

Alice, a strait-laced, perfectionist, and borderline saint, listened to him and talked him through it but knew she would not and could not prescribe oxycontin for this man. Instead, she ordered prescription-strength ibuprofen.

A few days after Christmas, we received service of process through certified mail from State B saying that Teladoc Inc., Teladoc PA, and Dr. Carol had broken the laws of this state. The documents explained how they would shut us down and Dr. Carol would lose her license. We were stunned! Was this a joke? Dr. Carol had written a prescription for ibuprofen, and this state was calling *that* a felony simply because she treated a patient she had never touched. I received a call from a sobbing Alice Carol, saying how this was going to ruin her life, and I assured her we would figure out a way to handle it.

I immediately picked up the phone and called the State B Board of Medical Examiners and asked, "Can Dr. Carol and I come out, meet with you, and talk through this?"

They agreed, and sometime in mid-January, we found ourselves in State B, sitting before the Board, telling our side of the story. They were not agreeable to it at first, so we hired a lawyer to advise us in that state and set up sessions where we could go in and tell our story under oath to try and find a solution or middle ground. I was really clear with our State B counsel that we did not want anything adversarial, so the better pathway would be to have him advise me, while we attended. I also brought in a high profile, well-known pediatrician who had cared for the children of two presidents while they were in the White House. That pediatrician had been a surgeon general candidate and was quite comfortable navigating difficult waters.

By mid-March, we were still at a stalemate and Dr. Carol was coming to these sessions, in tears, fearful of losing her license. Interestingly, she was continuing to donate her time to the state, and work in the reserves. One more important point: she was now five months pregnant! Paint that picture in your mind: pregnant saint crying while the Board was adamant about their perspective. At the time, I was convinced that State B's tactics and lack of concern for this great doctor was ruthless.

I believe it was the third session when State B made a mistake that turned the tides. While under oath, instead of referring to the man who had been prescribed ibuprofen by Dr. Carol as their patient, they called him their actor.

"Wait. Is he a patient, or is he an actor who works for the Board?" I asked for clarification.

We were under oath. Of course, they didn't want to answer that question! Nevertheless, they said it didn't matter because Dr. Carol had still treated a patient she hadn't touched, and that was a crime.

"Yes, but this looks like entrapment, and that is also a crime!" I declared.

They didn't seem to care.

That night in my hotel room, I was distraught about the situation. If they were willing to use their power to go to those extents, what else would they be willing to do? In my opinion, Dr. Carol is exactly the kind of person we want practicing medicine, and they were intent on destroying her career for ibuprofen!

I did something I had never done before. I called a local newspaper and let them know that State B had hired an actor in an apparent attempt to trick doctors into "committing a crime." The Board's tactic wasn't just a request for meds, it was a crying man using Christmas holidays as part of his tool.

He was not in pain! He was deliberately acting to entrap Dr. Carol. The newspaper did an article on the case and a few others and the State B Board of Medical Examiners promptly dropped the charge that would have taken Dr. Carol's license (with a possible prison term) and sanctioned her instead.

State B allowed cross coverage but limited any prescription to five days. The medical issue with that piece of code is that a proper term of antibiotics is ten days. Essentially, the state was forcing a covering doctor to commit medical malpractice in the event of an infection treated by a ten-day antibiotic. The legislation was already controversial in the medical community.

Dr. Carol had written the ibuprofen script for more than five days, and that became The Board's claim. The punishment for that was a simple letter. Within a few years, everything changed in State B, and they adopted telemedicine as a viable service in their state.

In my mind, Dr. Carol is one of the heroes of the telemedicine revolution. I hope her career has paid her the successful dividends she deserves.

State C

The functional lead for Teladoc PA, was Dr. John Marlowe (name changed), who was also an Eagle Scout and Navy Lieutenant. After we created the SuperDoc program, we started to get Dr. Marlowe licensed in many states. In the process of getting him licensed in State C, the state reached out to us stating that they needed us to report to their Board of Medical Examiners on a certain date and to explain what Dr. Marlowe was planning to do with his license in State C. They expressed an interest with a request that we elaborate more on our telemedicine company. After some research, I realized that State C had shut down several other physicians who were trying to practice telemedicine in the state.

I called the US senator for State C, who was also a medical doctor, and asked if he could help us. He told me no. He said that even though he was a US senator, he believed they would take *his* license if he associated with a telemedicine company! However, he wished us luck and told me to call him afterwards and let him know how it went.

Again, I was joined in this meeting by the same high-profile pediatrician/Surgeon General candidate who came with us to the State B sessions. We'll call him Dr. Atticus Lee. Dr. Lee suggested we go early to get a sense for how the Board of State C works, so the two of us traveled there together. We spent the morning watching the physicians in the state who had lost their licenses, and come in to make a case for why they should get them back.

Each session would begin with an explanation of the crime or violation committed by the doctor that had caused the state to suspend their license. Then, the doctor would explain what they had been doing in the interim, then make a case for why they should get their license back. It was a rather shocking day! Some of the mistakes were simple, but some were significant. I remember that one physician had inappropriate sexual contact with one of his patients. Another had been suspended for over-prescribing pain killers, and one was even abusing the pain killers himself! It was interesting to me that many of these doctors were doing morally reprehensible things, and yet, every single one of them got back their license by the end of the day. I am not arguing the logic of the State C Board. They know their protocols and rules and how to apply them. I am certain they were doing what made sense for their state.

Dr. Marlowe arrived about twenty minutes before his session, and by that time, we were thinking, this is a no brainer! We've got an Eagle Scout, Navy officer. All he is wants to do is telemedicine. This should go well for us!

We told our story. The Board of State C interrogated us harshly, and in the end, they told us, "No. We will not grant Dr. Marlowe his license in State C."

There was no crime committed because Dr. Marlowe had not done any consults, but the Board wanted to hear what we were doing with telemedicine before they were going to grant him his license in the state. We were astounded that, in this state, they would give licenses back to sexual abusers, doctors over-prescribing narcotics, and doctors addicted to narcotics...and yet they were telling an Eagle Scout, Navy lieutenant physician who merely wanted to practice telemedicine, "No."

This took place in late 2006 through early 2007. Interestingly, by this time, Dr. Sanders had already introduced telemedicine to the medical school in this state and they were using it! Under the umbrella of a state-run body, telemedicine was accepted. Those of us who were out in the free market were taking the heat!

State D

The head of the company, which was one of our largest customers at the time, Tom Steinbeck (name changed), was very concerned about potential state issues. A few of our patients had their prescriptions flagged, and we received a call from the Board of Medical Examiners in State D. Tom, urging us to get this ironed out, connected me with the attorney general from the state, Jo Laurence (name changed). I called her and described Teladoc and what we were doing. Jo thought we were cutting edge and believed the State Legislature would endorse it. She invited me out to State D to present to her team.

At the end of the visit, we were asked to work with a representative recommended by the AG's office to write a piece of legislation. That process was fantastic! I had the opportunity to write my first Bill, which was soon to become one of the laws defining telemedicine the way Teladoc was doing it. Incidentally, by then, we had significant competition around the country. One of those competitors that I am aware of was a fairly large company based in State D.

State E

Donald Benson (name changed), the CEO of one of the largest county hospitals in America was underwater because so many locals were using the ER as a primary care facility, then not paying the bill. The ER was always crowded with sometimes a 5-hour wait! Donald and I developed a strategy to place a cubicle in the ER and tell people, they could wait the five hours, but if they had a minor issue an wanted faster care, they could use this new telemedicine service.

The program was a huge success. The ER wait shortened, and the hospital replaced expensive ER write-offs with lower telemedicine costs...until Benson's Board informed him that telemedicine was illegal and unethical.

The program was scrapped after a few very successful months.

A Visit from the Drug Enforcement Agency (DEA)

Sometime in 2006, I was sitting at my desk in a meeting when Ruthie Smith, my administrative assistant, came in to inform me I was needed up front. Ruthie was absolute perfection all the time, and never would have interrupted me when I was in a meeting, so when she did, I knew something was wrong!

"I'm in a meeting," I said. "Can it wait?"

She then whispered in my ear, "The DEA is here...and they have their guns and badges."

That is one of the best reasons I have ever heard for ending a meeting...or maybe the worst!

I immediately left my office and found three officers waiting in our conference room displaying badges, and yes, fully armed. They had made quite a ruckus, so everyone in the building knew they were there. I sat down across from them, trying to be my normal, eternal-optimist self, and ask them what I could do for them.

"We have it on a good source that your company is writing prescriptions for narcotics, and we are going to take this place apart until we find the truth." The lead investigator said.

"My team will help you 100%," I said, with relief. "I can tell you with absolute confidence that no such thing was occurring. We intentionally built safeguards to prevent any narcotics from being prescribed."

This was one of the things Dr. Brooks, Begia and

Moczygemba had been adamant about. Telemedicine is not a tool for diagnosing things that require narcotics. It should never be a delivery mechanism to prescriptions of controlled substances.

We had an excellent system in place where strict rules were defined in the physician training. In addition, doctors were not allowed under our system to call in a prescription for the patient. For a host of reasons, we hired a team of nurses whose job was to review all the physician's notes, and then call in any prescription for the doctor.

We felt like this had been a foolproof system. I explained that it should have been close to impossible for a prescription for a narcotic to slip by unnoticed.

"We will see." The DEA was not convinced.

For three next three months, we worked with them as they investigated every computer file and printed file both at Teladoc, Inc. and down in San Antonio at Teladoc, PA. Many of our doctors and all our nurses were interrogated. In the end, the DEA found nothing.

Something like this can be disruptive for the staff, but our team remained positive and responsive to all of the requests made by the DEA officers.

The happy ending to this story is that, at the completion of their investigation, the DEA saw the value that Teladoc could bring them, as many DEA officers were traveling for work frequently and often not in their home state when they were sick. The officers who worked on our case ended up becoming Teladoc members and used the service!

The underlying theme in these stories is that we were convinced the only way to win the war was to do so without the fight. I didn't want to win through lawyers, guns, and money—I wanted to win through thought leadership. We wrote dozens of articles and white papers. We gave speeches, met with politicians and corporate leaders.

In December 2007, we celebrated our millionth member under the Rotunda in the US Capital Building. Our first major customer, Joel Ray, from New Benefits, attended, along with our millionth member. Former HHS Secretary Tommy Thompson officiated along with Newt Gingrich, Congresswoman Barbara Lee, and Senator Tom Coburn. In attendance were several other well-known politicians, corporate CEOs, and dignitaries.

During all that celebration, I was still co-processing on several states that were adamantly opposing the now tidal wave of telemedicine. By 2007, we had dozens of competitors, some doing it right, others not so careful. I was never too worried about the little ones. For me, the fun part was seeing all of the new companies that had names derived from Teladoc, like Phone-A-Doc, ConsultADoc and DialADoc.

Around that time, a company was started that I knew was going to be successful. At the time, we had raised less than $5 million—in total! This new company was purported to have raised over seven times that. I asked Ruthie to find a phone number and connect me. One of the most interesting conversations of my time at Teladoc happened on that call.

The founder of that company was suspicious from the start of the call.

"What do you want?" he asked.

I explained how we had been doing this for a very long time, and it was important for those of us who were considered the leaders, to do it right. We needed to recognize the laws of the 50 states, and strictly adhere to them.

He listened.

"There are a lot of companies trying to do telemedicine, and until now, we did not really have a serious competitor," I explained to him, "so welcome to the competition."

"Buddy," he paused for effect, "this is not a competition you can win. We will crush you so hard and so fast that no one will even remember the name Teladoc."

I swear, I cannot remember his name.

Fun, right?

In the course of my term at Teladoc, we received certified mail and service of process from the Boards of Medical Examiners of seventeen states. Each time, they suggested we bring a lawyer, but we almost never did, because we didn't want to make it into a legal battle. We always told them we simply wanted to improve medicine in their state. Instead of lawyers, we brought in thought leaders who sometimes were involved in telemedicine, and sometimes were not. Jay Sanders was a huge resource and often one of the ones we brought during this time!

We felt like every state was different, so we individually researched, called friends, and found every person who we thought would be an influencer or thought leader to the Boards. I admit, I had some sleepless nights!

When I knew I had to go present to a Board, I would think about who might be most beneficial to bring along. I would even do research on every board member in that state! I would know their hobbies, where they grew up, where they went to medical school, or if they were lawyers, where they went to law school. When I got into that room to present, I could usually look at each one of them and know their background. I spent so much of my time making sure that when we went into those meetings, we weren't going to have a negative situation.

Sometimes Board members wanted to be confrontational, but I always made sure they knew that we just wanted to improve medicine! Often, they would make requests, and we would jump through the hoops to fulfill those.

Post Moon Landing - Teladoc

By the summer of 2008, I was feeling pretty good about the trajectory. I was fond of saying that we had a couple million members to whom we were delivering doctors in about twelve minutes for $35. It was quite the claim!

A fun side story—Buzz Aldrin, who walked on the Moon with Neil Armstrong in 1969, had become an advisor and friend of the company. Buzz opened a lot of doors for us and added to the inspiration that my team exhibited every day. Imagine having someone who the history books will forever remember, coming into the office to talk to the team. I think most of the employees from that time period still treasure their photo and time with Buzz. For my own part, I know that his name recognition and ability to open doors played a defined role in our early success. I believe this is a valuable lesson to the entrepreneurs reading this book.

Most importantly, I was also beginning to realize that Teladoc had grown to the point where we needed a CEO who understood healthcare far better than me. John Halsey, and many others around me were incredible knowledge resources, but every successful entrepreneur should know their starting point and ending point.

After some interviews, Jason Gorevic was the obvious choice. In the summer of 2009, I handed over the baton. It was both a happy and a sad moment. Jason and his team have had a few issues that I am aware of, but the company always prevailed in the end. Another important lesson for entrepreneurs is to know your starting point and ending point in the journey of a company. I personally give Jason great credit for bringing the company as far as it has come.

As entrepreneurs, we think of our startups like children. A few years ago, I told a member of the press that Jason had "married my daughter" and was a good husband. That reporter did not get the analogy and responded, "How convenient for you!"

In July 2016, MIT Technology Review named Teladoc as one of the 50 Smartest companies in the World. My kids were fond of pointing out that we beat companies like Microsoft, IBM, Facebook, and Uber. Not bad, considering ten years earlier we were trying to make sure we didn't all go to prison!

In the beginning, and now, Dr. Sanders is planting the seeds and carrying the torch.

Hey, guess what, Jay? You should be proud—the rocket has reached orbit, and we have walked on the Moon!

Jay Sanders, the man who is the true father of telemedicine, is now in his mid-80s. It has been the great fortune of the Teladoc and now Recuro teams to have him onboard as an advisor and friend. Jay is still one of the great innovators who has a vision for what is next. He and I always joke around that if he is the father of telemedicine, then he is my father. …and dad to a lot of others like me, out there.

Another one of the great healthcare innovators of our time is Michael Brombach, who I have the pleasure of working with at Recuro. In the final chapter, we will combine the creativity of three generations, from Jay Sanders to me, to Michael Brombach. This group, spanning fifty years of age, will paint the picture for what is next.

CHAPTER 9

Sanders, Gorton, Brombach

From Efficiency of Telemedicine to Complete Care

The only way to discover the limits of the possible, is to
venture a little way past them, to the impossible.
— Arthur C. Clark

This book began with the *Butterfly Effect*. Patient Nelson would likely have died that day. Instead, he became a perfect case study for a new version of efficient care. On that day, Dr. Brooks' advice convinced Nelson to go to the ER. The historic pathway to that consultation can be traced back to the day Ken Bird, MD, first proposed treating patients using TV cameras. On that day, Dr. Sanders thought he was nuts.

With time, Jay Sanders, MD, became the torch-carrying advocate. Over his career, he would pass up opportunities in places like Iran and the Philippines, but he introduced telemedicine into prisons, state governments, and the Department of Defense. His evangelism led him to the University of Texas Medical Branch in Galveston where he met Oscar Boultinghouse, MD.

When the Texas Legislature mandated that incarcerated individuals receive care within 24 hours of their request, it seemed impossible. But Dr. Boultinghouse, with the technical assistance of Dr. Brooks, found a way.

It is impossible to know how many people have been positively impacted by the Butterfly Effect that occurred in the Summer of 1967. At the beginning of COVID, Michael Gorton received an email from one of the prior Surgeons General, recognizing the efforts and thanking him for the persistence that finally gave doctors the ability to efficiently and remotely see patients during lockdown. That number of telemedicine consultations has easily grown into hundreds of millions.

That was the Butterfly Effect of 1967. Until now, that has been the topic of this book, but something bigger is on the horizon.

Much bigger.

With the delivery engine in full force, how will that Telemedicine Revolution impact what is next?

Along with the founding of Teladoc, Dr. Brooks and Michael Gorton created a guarantee that a doctor would call the patient within three hours, or it was free. The accounting team was terrified that the company would be giving away a lot of free consults. That did not happen. The engine worked and within a few years of founding the company, Teladoc's doctors were treating patients within 12 minutes, nationwide.

These days, it is commonplace for a telemedicine provider to see a patient in less than 10 minutes of the initial request. Against all odds, the thousands of people who built the telemedicine industry, worked with determination and grit, and ultimately improved delivery in the practice of medicine.

Despite this, what we accomplished at Teladoc was

little more than a new efficiency paradigm for the conventional, existing reactive care system. The term reactive means people generally don't see their doctor until they are sick. The entire healthcare system is mostly reactive.

Think about it, the system is designed to do almost nothing until the patient is sick. Shouldn't we more accurately call it a "sick care system?"

A few years ago, Michael Gorton began thinking about how we could revolutionize healthcare again and make it preemptive. He called John Halsey and posed the questions: How can we catch things before they become dangerous and expensive? How can we minimize the number of situations where people are not feeling well, visit their doctor, and get a stage four cancer diagnosis?

Is there a solution?

Decades after the founding of Teladoc, healthcare costs have continued to rise every year. And yet, people continue to get diagnoses for maladies they might have been able to preempt.

Those of us who created and built Teladoc think of her as a child, but that child has grown up and is now married and living on her own. Teladoc has become an important model in our care system, but we, the innovators, cannot fix the fundamental broken parts of the care system with Teladoc.

Because of that, a new team consisting of Gorton, Halsey, Brombach, Allison Martin, Kim Darling, William Paiva, Drew Holm, Gina Fioretti and dozens of others came together to build an entirely new engine that would do tele-medicine better than Teladoc and add the next generation of tools specifically designed to catch medical issues before they become dangerous and expensive.

The goal of Recuro Health and this new engine should not just impact annual rising costs, but more importantly, it should lower them. This new preemptive approach will keep people healthier, with a long-term goal of increasing health-span and longevity.

How it is Done

The end product of the healthcare delivery system of tomorrow needs to recognize that simplicity and access are critical elements of the solution. The engine we have developed is already delivering a new generation of precision medicine. The best news is that we see tremendous innovation in both the short term and long term that will continue the acceleration.

What do we mean by precision medicine? If you Google it, you will find a narrow definition that uses genomics and other similar tools. This is just the beginning.

Let's say a woman named Greta goes in for her annual physical. The nurse checks her blood pressure, and it's 90/50. That number is entered into the medical record. That's a great number and very normal for Greta, as for anyone her age. The doctor comes in, reviews it, and tells her she looks great.

The next year when Greta goes in for her physical, her

blood pressure is 100/60. Again, it is a perfectly normal number for her age group. The doctor tells her she's healthy.

The third year, Greta returns, and her blood pressure is 110/70. The doctor tells her she's healthy; she's well within the normal range.

Greta is concerned because she notices that her blood pressure has been trending up, but the doctor, seeing a static number, perfectly normal for a woman her age, tells her she is well. Anything below 120/80 is considered healthy—but is it healthy for Greta?

Even though 110/70 blood pressure would be considered a normal number. With precision medicine, it would have been flagged for the physician by artificial intelligence (AI) built into the medical record.

This is a critical point. The medical record is a file and is static. It seldom shows trend lines. In Greta's case, there was an increase in the last two readings. By themselves, they are not red flags. As a trend line, they might be.

If the trend is flagged, perhaps the physician would approach it with more curiosity. Why was her blood pressure increasing every year? Was she stressed? Does she have a family history of high blood pressure? How are her calcium, magnesium, and potassium levels? Was she appropriately hydrated? What is her blood pressure like at other times of the day?

We now have the ability to radically change the medical record and overall way we collect, analyze, and use information to better inform patient care. We did this once when we introduced the Electronic Medical Record (EMR). Prior to the EMR, a medical record was a paper file, locked in a cabinet in the doctor's office. While the electronic version has taken a long time from its inception to viability, we now have the technology to deliver it anywhere, anytime.

We have the technology, but implementation is lagging. The next step is the introduction of a dynamic data engine and integrated care platform or Digital Medical Home, a new concept trademarked by Recuro Health. The Digital Medical Home (DMH) is not a static snapshot updated with the doctor visit, but a living platform that can be fed the right data continuously to enable a care team to provide the next generation of healthcare. As that data is fed into the DMH, Artificial Intelligence (AI) can monitor and watch for unusual blips, suggest interventions, coordinate care outreach, and support clinical decision making.

On a side note, the term Digital Medical Home was coined by John Halsey, and in the beginning, trademarked by Recuro. In recent months, we have chosen to relax that trademark It is an obvious term, and a perfect descriptor that should be used by any person or company interested in using it.

One of the great realizations of the telemedicine revolution should be that the DMH belongs to the patient, not the doctor, and as such, goes wherever the patient is. The implications go way beyond the simple storage of data to a dynamic resource that contributes to the patient's daily health. It provides actionable guidance and supports the patient throughout the entire care journey with personalized treatment. For all those who have been frustrated by filling out the same paperwork every time they enter a new medical facility, the DMH is the answer.

It should be noted that the DMH would not have been possible during the early days at Teladoc. It is now possible because of tools like the Microsoft Cloud for Healthcare. Using these tools, companies like Recuro can accelerate transformation by augmenting the Microsoft Cloud with industry relevant compliance, security, and interoperability standards. It helps unifying the data estate through a common data model to break down data silos, helping organizations improve insights, regardless of where the data resides.

The key is: "regardless of where the data resides." It should be accessible from anywhere, and the cloud provides that kind of access. As Dr. Sanders reiterated when he treated an allergy patient sitting on an old chair, with a cat in her lap and a cigarette smoking husband behind her—whenever practicable, the patient should be treated wherever they happen to be, not in the doctor's office.

As we continue to implement remote patient monitoring, Greta would have home devices capturing data and delivering her blood pressure, temperature, pulse rate and other vital signs—along with a time stamp. Already, there are wearable devices, like the Apple Watch, Aura Ring, and dozens of similar pieces of technology which are constantly picking up a person's pulse, blood oxygen level, heart rhythm, and more. In the future, these devices will even use optics to test blood glucose and, using micro-needle technology, interstitial fluid. Instead of the current norm where people go to the doctor only once a year, these devices could be sending megabits of data with her vital signs to her DMH continuously. The AI algorithms would alert the PCP, care team, or the patient if something unusual popped up. The data could easily be shown in the form of trendline graphs.

As we enter a new age of continuous data, scientists and physicians will begin to use the trendlines from that data to detect and even avert early onset of disease and medical issues that are currently wrecking lives and costing millions of dollars

The power of this cannot be understated. Tiny changes, based on health risk assessments, when analyzed by a processor that can handle trillions of instructions per second, can be sent to a doctor for further review. Medical records stored in data structures like the Microsoft Cloud can be instantaneously available to any provider, anywhere.

The ability to collect and analyze data for the willing patient already exists everywhere around us.

One location where it might make perfect sense to implement sensor technology for remote patient monitoring is the personal automobile! When a person gets into their car and turns on the ignition, everything lights up and they instantly have all the information they could possibly need regarding the status of their car—tire pressure, whether the oil needs changed, how much fuel is in the tank, and more. However, there is no information on the most important thing in the car—the driver.

When a person sits down in the driver's seat, their weight could be recorded. When they put their hands on the steering wheel, their rhythm strip, pulse, and pulse oximetry could be obtained. When the seatbelt is stretched across the driver's chest and plugged in, their respiratory rate and volume could be detected.

Imagine a dashboard that tells you not only everything about the car, but everything you could possibly need to know about the driver! Imagine that a person gets in a car accident and immediately, the car can send their most up-to-date vital signs to the EMT enroute in the ambulance. Their most current healthcare information and pre-existing conditions are already available to the EMTs, doctors, and nurses in the patients DMH, which has been continuously creating trend lines for hours, weeks, or possibly years.

Another obvious place is the bed where you sleep every night. Several innovations by companies like Matteo Franceschetti's Eight Sleep mattress cover can capture relevant data every time you go to bed. That data will be fed into a DMH to be analyzed and sorted with AI, then graphed for your medical provider.

Additionally, we believe the artificial intelligence system will be programmed to the individual patient's genetic makeup that may catch the more subtle shifts even quicker than a busy physician could.

It is important to clarify that this represents a tool to be utilized by the doctor, not a replacement for that doctor.

As the creators of the industry, we are confident in the prediction that telemedicine, as we now know it, will NOT play a significant part in evolving the future of medicine. Telemedicine is just an efficiency tool that improves the delivery of care.

When a patient calls a doctor, she is getting a diagnosis based on the specific knowledge base and education of that one doctor, for better or for worse. With the implementation of improved clinical decision support and artificial intelligence, which can draw upon a worldwide web of the most up-to-date research, studies, and medical textbooks, physicians have the most relevant information possible to diagnose and treat a patient.

Artificial intelligence would have the capability of interrogating the patient's DMH in real time with the diagnostic criteria entered by the physician, the signs and symptoms, and the prescribed medications against the best literature in the world related to that diagnosis. It would then alert the physician if they were doing anything that was contraindicated or clue them in if there was a more proven way to treat that patient. The physician of the future will be more like the conductor of a full symphony with an entire world of musician-medicine at her fingertips for diagnosis and treatment.

Artificial intelligence would have the capability of interrogating the patient's DMH in real time with the diagnostic criteria entered by the physician, the signs and symptoms, and the prescribed medications against the best literature in the world related to that diagnosis. It would then alert the physician if they were doing anything that was contraindicated or clue them in if there was a more proven or innovative method to treat that patient.

A Johns Hopkins study published in 2016 stated that medical errors in the United States account for more than 250,000 deaths per year. This would make a medical error the third leading cause of death in the United States behind only heart disease and cancer. In the future, artificial intelligence could significantly reduce this number due to its ability to alert the physician of the most up-to-date research and best practices. With AI, millions of data points can be used in every diagnosis and treatment.

As Doctor Sanders learned in 1995 when he did that first house-call using a patient's home television, the exam room needs to be where the patient lives, not where the doctor works. Remote patient monitoring, artificial intelligence, integrated care teams and a DMH will make that more possible than ever before. These technologies would also give us the power to take our health into our own hands. We could have the information flow that would clue us in to a potential issue before it becomes dangerous. The healthcare delivery system would be there to help us stay healthy, not fix us after we are sick.

New Methods and Technologies

Can technology fix the biggest problems in healthcare?

Not by itself. But technology can create patient empowerment and enhanced personalization. It can give the patient and provider the right tools, data, and access to do more for their own healthcare. If delivered with simplicity, technology can help to pave the road. There are still issues that are too complex for an average person to figure out on their own that will require the healthcare delivery system to help them "fix it."

Traditional telehealth solved a convenience problem, solved a patient access problem, and partially solved an affordability problem. Ultimately, it was designed to take care services exactly as they were and extend them to wherever the patient happened to be.

With telemedicine, the care model did not change.

Virtual care delivery as a technology is no more than an enabler for the existing, reactive healthcare system. If we really want to address the problems we need to solve in the future, we are going to have to modify the type of care we deliver in system. To reiterate the point, we believe that telemedicine is only relevant to the discussion as an efficient and scalable platform for care delivery.

The *type* of care we are delivering must change.

First, we need to blend the physical with the remote—traditional with telemedicine.

Second, we need to broaden the preemptive aspects.

Preemptive, hyper-personalized and proactive medicine are the best pathways to lowering costs and keeping people healthy.

To become preemptive and correctly deliver care, a more complete picture is needed than what we currently have in healthcare.

The beginning foundation must be built on a solid and thorough health risk assessment. Accomplishing this objective requires that we understand the genetic and epigenetic factors that impact an individual's health.

Epigenetics is the study of how the environment and your behavior influences the workings of your genes. In other words, what you eat, how you act, what you drink, and where you live can influence your gene expression. A very simple example of epigenetics is a florist changing the color of a flower with dyed water. Science is discovering much more complex examples that will impact health and longevity in humans.

Once we build the foundation with risk assessment, genomics and environmental factors, we need a continuous stream of data. Remote patient monitoring will deliver a huge piece of that data.

For clarity, the historic definition of the word *patient* would mean someone who is sick, but now it should be broadened to mean everyone—sick or healthy. When Joey puts on his Apple Watch every day, he does so to utilize the tool. That tool should collect data that gets transferred to the Digital Medical Home. That is Remote Patient Monitoring (RPM)

The Apple Watch is a single example of the hundreds of data collection devices we will use to capture data that can help keep people healthy. The number of new tools is growing and will continue to grow on a regular basis.

A half-dozen years ago, a young South African entrepreneur named Allison Martin came to the US to build a company that would simplify delivery of labs into the home. This reiterated Dr. Sander's thesis that care should be brought to the patient.

To create a complete picture, we must include alternative data sets like environmental influencers, social determinants of health, sleep monitoring, exercise, life cycle data, and remote labs. All these items should be captured continuously and added to the Digital Medical Home.

With all this information, we have a baseline, from which we can now calculate potential risk factors. If the data suggests someone is at risk for heart disease, we should preemptively test and watch for the signs. Because we have analysis and probabilities, it makes sense to send a test into the home. For clarity, a home lab is far less detrimental or expensive than a heart attack!

For Complete Care, we evaluate all the science, biochemistry, genetics, epigenetics, diagnostic labs, and historical information. When compiled, all these resources create the workings of an incredibly accurate personalized patient profile.

A true DMH should be accumulating far more data than any provider could assess. That is why the next critical element is the data engine, constantly monitoring the flow of information for anomalies.

The artificial intelligence engine will catch every trend line that has potential negative repercussions. It has been taught the best practices and protocols. As Jay Sanders mentioned, what's wrong with the patient will be flagged against the best data that's out there for the protocols to treat their specific ailment or issue. The data goes to the doctor, and that doctor now has the best tools to make informed decisions.

There will be plenty of cases where individuals choose not to use the tools to support their proactive care. It could very well seem scary to have your biometric and health data constantly feeding a dynamic health profile in the DMH. For some, it will seem like "Big Brother" from George Orwell's dystopian novel, 1984.

Medical records are designed to be one of the most secure data structures in existence. For those who recognize this, passing data to a DMH will be an easy decision. For those who lack the trust, it could be a scary proposition. This of course, will be one of the challenges to adoption.

Next Steps

We can spend a lot of time developing the tools, technology and biochemistry to keep people healthy. Mathematics and science are adopting the analytics tools and computing engines to predict the future. With AI, we are actually developing intelligence in our machines to evaluate, make conclusions, and sometimes respond.

With all of this, there is one important element that no amount of technology can replace.

The touch and feel of humanity.

As we develop the decision support tools, we must always remember that, in the end, a caring and knowledgeable physician, utilizing the best tools of the day, will prevail against even the best AI and analytics engines that do not have a human interface.

The goal of these authors, and of our company Recuro Health, is to catch and treat things before they get expensive and dangerous. Healthcare costs continue to increase every year. Our friends and family are still receiving dangerous diagnoses that technology and proper care could catch.

Our mission is to solve this problem.

How can we be proactive and change the way medicine operates now? At Recuro, we have built the first generation of an engine that is beginning to accomplish that goal. Admittedly, we have a long way to go.

We learned while building Teladoc that even the best solutions take time for adoption. We also learned that simplicity is the best path to crossing the finish line and reaching the populace.

Recuro has begun by building what we believe is the best telemedicine engine in existence today. Recognizing that every telehealth company says that; we fall back on the credibility that Jay Sanders is the Father of Telemedicine, and we did in fact build the first great telemedicine delivery engine!

With the delivery platform (aka, the best tech enabled telemedicine engine!), we can continue to simplify and introduce the preemptive elements. Adoption is slow but increasing, and we have become the thought leaders and evangelists.

In the early years of the Internet, I (Michael Gorton) would give talks at the Rotary, Chambers of Commerce, and anyone who would let me speak. Today, it is difficult to imagine a time when people did not know what the Internet was. Back then, no one did! I would talk about things like email addresses and the world wide web. Some people thought I was a kook, but ultimately, it became mainstream, just like Teladoc. Thought leadership, speeches, white papers, books, and articles were the elements that created the avalanche.

Another clever way to accelerate the process would be to gamify the patient's healthcare! I think Delta and American Airlines have done a great job of gamifying airline status. For American Airlines, Executive Platinum is the pinnacle status. To achieve it, you almost never purchase a ticket on a competitor airline. It is a simple and straightforward goal, gamified with success plateaus.

For healthcare, let's imagine a scenario where Susan has a Digital Medical Home. Every time there is an abnormal blip in her data, the provider calls and makes a suggestion or modification to her daily activities. Susan implements those suggestions because they are simple and straightforward. The data then shows her corrected behavior and an improvement in her overall health. Now, introduce an actuary—a mathematical genius who knows how to calculate probability. The actuary runs an analysis of Susan and realizes that she is willing and able to modify behavior based on the new Complete Care engine.

Susan gets a phone call from her insurance company: "Susan, we have noticed that you are willing to do what is necessary to maintain your health. Because of this, your insurance premium will be dropping this year. Keep it up, and your premium will continue to drop."

That's right, we did use the term "dropping" as it applies to healthcare costs! Are you having an out-of-body reaction to that one?

Susan tells her friends and family about how her insurance company has gamified her insurance—like becoming a member of the American Airlines Executive Platinum Program. Susan is now more determined than ever to continue the trend.

Those of us who are creating, building, and delivering the next generation of healthcare must recognize that our real job is to prevent first, and treat when necessary. Our responsibility is significant and to effectively accomplish this goal, we must simplify everything that touches the patient.

We often use the analogy that almost no one runs out

of gas on the side of the road. Why is that? While internal combustion engines are complex machines with thousands of moving parts, we have made driving them—simple. We don't run out of gas because we have a gas gauge.

We don't have a gas gauge equivalent for our body.

Yet.

That is all about to change.

Health and Longevity

As patients, we need to learn to use the human form of the automobile gas gauge. Our next generation of Digital Medical Home and Complete Care will let us know when it is time to "fill up."

The human immune system, in many ways, is still the best medicine in existence. Keeping it strong and not over-burdened should be one of the objectives of a preemptive system. Science and medicine are discovering the best ways to do just that. This book is not being written as a medical guide, so we will leave the specifics to the health-care providers.

What we know is that there is a close correlation between the things we need to do regularly to stay healthy, and the things we should do to increase the number of years we stay healthy and strong, also known as our healthspan.

Mom taught us many of those things. Eat healthy meals, exercise regularly and take our vitamins. Science is showing us that we have food allergies, and as such, things to avoid. Genomics panels can help us understand which drugs are effective, and which aren't. Sometimes, which are dangerous.

We are coming to an age of individualized medicine. There is an old nursery rhyme: *Jack Spratt could eat no fat. His wife could eat no lean.* So, between the two of them, they'd lick the platter clean. Husband and wife—completely different metabolisms.

Soon, we will have great clarity on what we can and should put in our bodies as individuals. Genomics will give us some of this. Most of us have grown up on standardized portions, vitamin amounts, rest and exercise. Over the next twenty years, those standards will become very individualized.

Jeff Gladden, MD, is one of the preeminent longevity physicians today. Dr. Gladden is working to deliver a science where age 100 will be the new 30. Gladden is fond of saying that we will get to the point where, at 100, we will look and feel like we did at 30.

One of our objectives is to help him deliver on that promise. We recognize like any great achievement in life, it probably won't happen with a magic pill. We will need to study, work, play, exercise, eat right, and make good decisions to maintain our health at that level for that long.

Thomas Edison once said:

The doctor of the future will give no medicine but will instead instruct patients in the care of the human frame, in diet, and in the cause of prevention of disease.

Wow, a century ago, Edison predicted it. We agree.

For Nelson, who started out this book with the *Butterfly Effect* from 1967, we say there will be millions more, who like Nelson, will prevail, as those of us in the healthcare industry come together to create the next generation of preemptive care.

Epilogue
by
Dr. Fab Mancini

Reading Digital Medical Home is like seeing the evolution of healthcare with a very clear lens. In the beginning of the book, the authors tell the (true) story of a man named Nelson who most likely survived a severe medical incident because he had access to telemedicine. As a doctor, author and speaker for the past 30 years, I am always looking for things that inspire, increase effectiveness, engage patient participation, and potentially change everything for the better. The content of this book will show the reader how telemedicine did exactly that. A year before the pandemic, very few people had ever heard of Teladoc. Now almost everyone has used it or a similar service. In a recent survey, most patients prefer telemedicine over a traditional doctor visit!

Telemedicine created a platform for delivery that changed the way we get care—worldwide. Before Teladoc, getting an appointment to see a doctor took days. Now, it is minutes. The idea was created by Harvard professor, Dr. Kenneth Bird, then brought to the world by his resident, Jay H. Sanders, MD, FACP. Teladoc, the first company to deliver telemedicine nationwide was founded by my friend and colleague, Michael Gorton.

Teladoc is an example of disruptive innovation. It is an

idea that changed everything, and launched, what is now a quarter trillion-dollar industry.

The real question is what's next?

Authors Sanders and Gorton address the "what's next?" question in the final chapter of this book. The next disruptive innovation is the Digital Medical Home, created by Recuro Health. The goal is three parts:

1. To deliver telemedicine better than any other company
2. To catch medical illness before they become serious
3. To empower the patient to become more knowledgeable and responsible for their own care

Proactive and preemptive care is the next generation of disruptive innovation. Sanders and Gorton, the authors of this book are thought leaders on a mission to fix the healthcare system, through their startup company Recuro Health, through public speeches, White Papers, and this book.

— Dr. Fab Mancini

America's #1 "Healthy Living" Media Expert, World Renowned Chiropractor, International Bestselling Author and Speaker, Business Consultant and President Emeritus of Parker University.

Michael S. Gorton, MS, JD

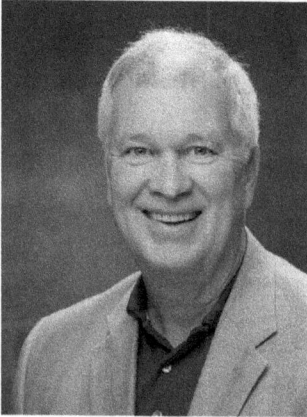

Mr. Gorton, co-founder of Recuro Health, is a 14-time Serial Entrepreneur and best-selling author whose companies have created industries, and tens of billions of dollars in wealth. He has experience building both public and private companies in the digital health, telecom, music, energy, healthcare, book publishing, aerospace, education and water remediation industries. Throughout his executive career, Michael has founded and led industry-changing companies, including Internet Global, Teladoc, Palo Duro Records, Principal Solar, Back To Space and Recuro Health. Michael is credited with being one of the pioneer/creators of the telemedicine industry, now approaching a half-trillion dollars globally. The Texas Business Hall of Fame has recently added Gorton to their Board. The World Economic Forum has named him a Tech Pioneer in healthcare, and Ernst and Young have named him Entrepreneur of the Year.

In 2021, Gorton and John Halsey along with some of the pioneers of telemedicine and digital health, created Recuro Health, a company that has developed a Digital Medical Home. Recuro now serves three million members with the next generation of care, delivered through brokers, TPA's and several of the Fortune Fifty companies. The Company has been recognized by the World Economic Forum as a Tech Pioneer in Healthcare, and by Ernst and Young as one of the nation's fasted growing companies.

As CEO, Chairman, and Founder of Teladoc, Gorton led a telemedicine company that was named by MIT as one of the Top 50 Smartest Companies in the World. Teladoc is now the world's leading telemedicine company with a NYSE market cap in the tens of billions of dollars. The digital and telemedicine industry, which Gorton helped to launch, is now approaching a half-trillion-dollar industry.

Gorton was the founding CEO of Principal Solar, a public company he led to become one of the thought leaders in the solar industry worldwide, that delivered 400 megawatts of sustainable electricity, enough to run approximately 70,000 American homes. With Internet Global, he led the company from concept to the #1 ranked Internet provider in North Texas and the construction of the world's first DSL network and one of the first national VOIP networks. He is currently starting a roll up in the telehealth and digital health industries, with a goal of fixing some of the major issues in healthcare today.

Michael studied physics and engineering at UT Austin and holds a JD in Law from Texas A&M University, a BS in Engineering from Texas Tech University, and an MS in Physics from The University of Texas. He serves on the Board of the Texas Business Hall of Fame, is a recipient of the coveted Ernst and Young Entrepreneur of the Year Award and is a World Economic Forum Tech Pioneer in Healthcare. Gorton is considered a thought leader with more than 30 white papers, 100+ articles, six novels and one business book on M&A transactions. His historic fiction novel *Forefathers and Founding Fathers* became an Amazon #1 best seller. Michael has run eighteen marathons, is working on his 3rd degree black belt in karate and has completed a 4,800-mile bicycle adventure across the US. He and his family have a goal of climbing the highest point of elevation in all 50 states. They have completed 42.

Michael S. Gorton
CEO and Founder

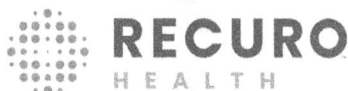

RECURO HEALTH

Recuro Health
https://recurohealth.com/

E-mail: mgorton@RecuroHealth.com
Telephone: (214) 923-1921

Jay H. Sanders, M.D., F.A.C.P., F.A.C.A.A.I., FATA

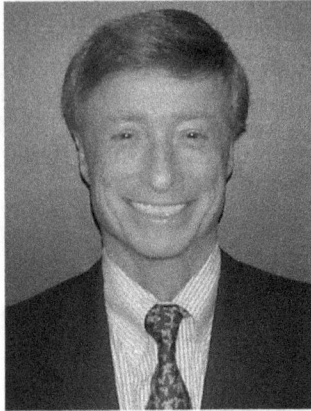

Jay H. Sanders, M.D. is President and CEO of The Global Telemedicine Group, Professor of Medicine at Johns Hopkins University School of Medicine (Adjunct), a Founding Board Member of the American Telemedicine Association where he serves as President Emeritus and headed the FCC's Rural Healthcare Fund and was the Scientific, Military and Medical Advisory Committee of the National Science Foundation ASSIST center developing medical sensors at North Carolina State University. He is identified by his colleagues as the "Father of Telemedicine".

Dr. Sanders has served on the NASA Biological and Physical Research Space Advisory Committee, as a consultant to the NASA Space Communication Center and was the Scientific Director for the NASA Medical Informatics and Technology Applications Commercial Space Center.

He has been a consultant to the Army's Telemedicine and Advanced Technology Research Center (TATRC) at Ft. Detrick, the CIO of the Military Healthcare System, the Defense Advanced Research Projects Agency (DARPA), the Air Force Center for Telehealth and Theater Informatics, the

Veteran Administration, and previously was appointed the only civilian member of the Department of Defense Telemedicine Board of Directors with the Surgeon Generals of the Army, Navy, and Air Force.

Dr. Sanders has served as a consultant to the Southern Governors' Homeland Security Telehealth Anti-Bioterrorism Task Force and was the Principal Investigator of a grant from the Office of the Secretary of Defense related to First Responder education and standards.

He was appointed by former Secretary of HHS, Michael Leavitt, to the Chronic Care Workgroup of the American Health Information Community Committee, and during the Clinton Administration he directed the U.S. telemedicine initiatives to the G-8 nations. Additionally, he has been a consultant to the World Health Organization on Health Telematics, as well as a consultant to the Russian Telemedicine Foundation.

He was a consultant to the MIT Media Lab, Vesalius Ventures, a Venture Capital Firm focusing on telehealth, medical informatics, and medical sensors and to Columbia University School of Medicine and their Center for Advanced Technology. He was formerly Visiting Professor at Yale University School of Medicine and Professor of Medicine and Surgery and Director of the Telemedicine Program at the Medical College of Georgia, where he held the Eminent Scholar Chair in Telemedicine. He headed the Medical Advisory Committee of the National Science Foundation—North Carolina State University ASSIST Nanosystems Center.

Dr. Sanders served as a member of the Executive Committee of the Board of Directors of the Federal Communications Commission Universal Service Administrative Corporation and was Chairman of its Rural Health Care Committee from its inception in 1996 to 2014. He served as a member of the National Library of Medicine's Long Range Planning Committee and as President and a member of the Executive Committee of the Board of Directors of the Friends of the National Library of Medicine.

He served on the Southern Governors Association Task Force on Medical Technology, the FCC Telemedicine Advisory Committee, and the Institute of Medicine/National Academy of Science Telemedicine Evaluation Committee.

Dr. Sanders earned his medical degree from Harvard Medical School Magna Cum Laude and was a member of AOA. He did his residency training at the Massachusetts General Hospital in Boston where he became Chief Medical Resident and did a research fellowship in Immunology at the National Institutes of Health. Following residency training, Dr. Sanders joined the University of Miami School of Medicine where he initiated the concept and established the first Division of General Medicine in the Department of Medicine in any Academic Medical Center. As Chief of that Division, he also headed the Medical Intensive Care Unit, the Medical House Staff Program and the Medical Division of the Emergency Department. He attained the rank of Professor of Medicine within six years after the completion of his Chief Residency and was Chief of Medicine at the University of Miami's Jackson Memorial Hospital, the largest teaching hospital in the Southeastern United States.

Dr. Sanders has spent the majority of his professional career involved in teaching, patient care and health care research. Identified by his colleagues as "the Father of Telemedicine" he has spent over 50 years in the development and implementation of telecommunications and information technologies as a means of addressing the problems relating to quality, cost and access to care that now plague our health care system. He was the Principal Investigator of a grant from the NSF that represented the first application of telemedicine into correctional healthcare, and in 1991 he designed the telemedicine system for the State of Georgia that interfaced with rural hospitals, public health facilities, correctional institutions, ambulatory health care centers, military bases and public-school classrooms. This was the first statewide telemedicine program in the country and served as the model for many other states to follow. He initiated a project at the Medical College of Georgia in 1993, in coordination with Georgia Tech where he had an appointment as Senior Research Scientist, that provided the first Tele-homecare technology application in the United States. Named the "Electronic House Call", the system allowed practitioners the ability to examine their patients over a cable TV interface in their homes, and the elderly in nursing homes. The author of numerous articles on telemedicine, he was an Associate Editor of the *Telemedicine and e-Health Journal* and has served on the editorial boards of the *Telemedicine Newsletter*, *Telemedicine Report*, *The Telemedicine Connection*, *Telemedicine and Telehealth Networks* and *Telemedicine and Virtual Reality*. He is also an editor of the book, *"Telemedicine: Theory and Practice"* a Charles C. Thomas publication. Dr. Sanders is a consultant for many academic, governmental, public and industrial organizations nationally and internationally.

Jay H. Sanders, M.D.
President and CEO
The Global Telemedicine Group

Telephone: (703) 448-9640
E-mail: jsanders@tgtg.com

Bibliography

Bird, Dr. Kenneth. 1991. *New York Times*—Used TV for diagnosis

https://www.nytimes.com/1991/02/16/obituaries/dr-kenneth-bird-73-used-tv-for-diagnosis.html

———

Davies, Dave. 2021. *NPR* - How the Attica prison uprising started and why it still resonates today

https://www.npr.org/2021/10/27/1049295683/attica-prison-documentary-stanley-nelson

———

Evon, Dan. 2022. *Snopes* - Was 'The Sound of Silence' inspired by Art Garfunkel's blind friend, Sandy Greenberg?

https://www.snopes.com/fact-check/art-garfunkel-sandy-greenberg/

———

Ferdinand Marcos. 2022. *Britannica* - Biography

https://www.britannica.com/biography/Ferdinand-E-Marcos

———

Gittelshon, John. 1991. *South Florida Sun Sentinel* - '69 dream homes lose original luster

https://www.sun-sentinel.com/news/fl-xpm-1991-03-31-9101160644-story.html

———

Golkar, Saeid and Sawhney, Asha. 2020. *Middle East Institute* - Dictators and civilizational thinking in Iran: From the Great Civilization to Islamic Civilization

https://www.mei.edu/publications/dictators-and-civilizational-thinking-iran-great-civilization-islamic-civilization#:~:text=Mohammad%20Reza%20Shah%20Pahlavi%20called,to%20completely%20emulate%20the%20West.

Johns Hopkins Medicine. 2016. Study suggests medical errors now third leading cause of death in the U.S.

https://www.hopkinsmedicine.org/news/media/releases/study_suggests_medical_errors_now_third_leading_cause_of_death_in_the_us

Ray, Michael. (n.d.) *Britannica* - Imelda Marcos. https://www.britannica.com/biography/Imelda-Marcos

Reverby, Susan M., PhD. 2018. *Sage Journals* - Can there be acceptable prison health care? Looking back on the 1970s.

https://journals.sagepub.com doi/10.1177/0033354918805985

Sanders, Jay, MD. 2018. *Med Page Today* - How 'a stupid idea' gave birth to telemedicine.

https://www.medpagetoday.com/practicemanagement/informationtechnology/55457

_____

Sosonowsky, Alex. (n.d.). *AccuWeather* - Why Florida ranks highest for lightning fatalities in the US. https://www.accuweather.com/en/weather-news/why-florida-ranks-highest-for-lightning-fatalities-in-the-us/350561

_____

Xie, Sunny. 2021. *China Highlights* - 10 interesting Yunnan facts for travelers https://www.chinahighlights.com/yunnan/yunnan-facts.htm

Special thanks to Sally Frank of Microsoft for providing language on Azure and the Microsoft Cloud.